Drug Stability for
Pharmaceutical Scientists

For her love and support this textbook is dedicated to my wife Hanna Lilja

Drug Stability for Pharmaceutical Scientists

Thorsteinn Loftsson

AMSTERDAM • BOSTON • HEIDELBERG • LONDON
NEW YORK • OXFORD • PARIS • SAN DIEGO
SAN FRANCISCO • SINGAPORE • SYDNEY • TOKYO
Academic Press is an imprint of Elsevier

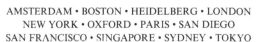

Academic Press is an imprint of Elsevier
The Boulevard, Langford Lane, Kidlington, Oxford, OX5 1GB, UK
225 Wyman Street, Waltham, MA 02451, USA

First published 2014

Notices
Knowledge and best practice in this field are constantly changing. As new research and experience broaden our understanding, changes in research methods, professional practices, or medical treatment may become necessary.

Practitioners and researchers must always rely on their own experience and knowledge in evaluating and using any information, methods, compounds, or experiments described herein. In using such information or methods they should be mindful of their own safety and the safety of others, including parties for whom they have a professional responsibility.

To the fullest extent of the law, neither the Publisher nor the authors, contributors, or editors, assume any liability for any injury and/or damage to persons or property as a matter of products liability, negligence or otherwise, or from any use or operation of any methods, products, instructions, or ideas contained in the material herein.

British Library Cataloguing in Publication Data
A catalogue record for this book is available from the British Library

Library of Congress Cataloging-in-Publication Data
A catalog record for this book is available from the Library of Congress

ISBN: 978-0-12-411548-4

For information on all Academic Press publications
visit our website at store.elsevier.com

This book has been manufactured using Print On Demand technology. Each copy is produced to order and is limited to black ink. The online version of this book will show color figures where appropriate.

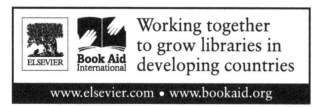

Working together
to grow libraries in
developing countries

www.elsevier.com • www.bookaid.org

CONTENTS

CHAPTER 1

Introduction

Stability of pharmaceutical products refers to the capacity of the product or a given drug substance to remain within established specifications of identity, potency, and purity during a specified time period. Drug stability can be divided into three categories: chemical stability, physical stability, and microbial stability (Table 1.1). Drug degradation can also be classified according to the environment created by the drug product (Table 1.2). The drug formulation can strongly influence the rate and mechanism of drug degradation. In general, drugs degrade at much faster rates in solution than in their solid states, and much faster in aqueous solutions than in no aqueous solutions. Besides monitoring the loss of the *active pharmaceutical ingredient* (API), (i.e., the drug), stability testing of a finished drug product may involve monitoring: formation of degradation products, changes in drug disintegration and dissolution, loss of package integrity, and microbial contamination. During stability testing of the finished drug product, the appearance of the product and its package will also be monitored. *Stability testing* provides evidence of how the quality of a finished drug product, API, or pharmaceutical excipient varies with time under the influence of a variety of environmental factors such as temperature, humidity, pH, and light. It can also provide evidence of how transportation, package materials, pharmaceutical excipients, and microbes affect the product. Stability testing of a finished drug product is performed under the guidelines of the *European Medicines Agency* (EMA), *Food and Drug Administration* (FDA), or some other authoritative organization. *Shelf-life* is the length of time the finished drug product will last without deteriorating. Frequently, shelf-life is defined as the time for the original potency (i.e., 100%) of the active drug to be reduced to 95% (t_{95}) or, more frequently, 90% (t_{90}), although more stringent time limits may apply if the degradation products are toxic. Besides chemical degradation of the active ingredient, the shelf-life can be limited by the physical stability of the drug products, such as changes in the drug crystal form or changes in the appearance of the drug product. Stability testing will provide information on the recommended storage

Table 1.1 The Three Main Categories of Drug Stability and Some Examples of Degradation Mechanisms

Category	Description	Examples
Chemical stability	Breakage or formation of covalent bonds resulting in, for example, loss of potency.	Ester hydrolysis
		Amide hydrolysis
		Lactam hydrolysis
		Oxidation
Physical stability	No breakage or formation of covalent bonds. Such changes can lead to changes in drug solubility or changes in the appearance of the drug product.	Crystallization of amorphous drugs
		Changes in crystal forms
		Loss of crystal water
Microbial stability	Microbial contamination	Aqueous eye drop solutions
		Parenteral solutions

Table 1.2 Classification of Drug Degradation According to the Drug Product Form

Form	Description	Examples
Solution	One liquid phase	Parenteral solutions
		Hydrogels
		Ointments
Suspension	One solid and one liquid phase	Oral suspensions
		Eye drop suspensions
Emulsion	Two liquid phases	Creams
Solid oral dosage form	One or more solid phases	Tablets, capsules

conditions, degradation products, and shelf-life of the drug product. The term *expiration date* (or *expiry date*) is sometimes defined as the date up until which the manufacturer guarantees the full safety and potency of the drug product. The expiration date may be set as a fixed time after product manufacturing, after dispensing of the product (e.g., oral antibiotic mixtures), or after opening the drug container (e.g., eye drops). Thus, the expiration date of a given drug product may differ from its shelf-life.

In chemistry, an *ideal solution* is defined as a solution whose activity coefficients are equal to unity. In such solutions, the interaction between molecules does not differ from the interactions between molecules of each component. In other words, an ideal solution is a solution that conforms exactly to Raoult's law. It shows no internal energy change on mixing and no attractive force between components. Pharmaceutical products are never ideal solutions and, thus, their physicochemical behavior can deviate from common theoretical equations and display unexpected behavior. Although various preformulation studies can be performed in dilute aqueous drug solutions, the final stability evaluations and shelf-life predictions have to be based on studies of the final pharmaceutical product.

Although drug degradation in the solid state is, in general, treated as a special case, it frequently follows the same degradation mechanisms as drug degradation in concentrated aqueous solutions. In such cases, the drug degradation rate may be proportional to the amount of water absorbed into the product.

CHAPTER 2

Principles of Drug Degradation

The rate of reaction may be defined as the rate of concentration changes of the reactants or products:

$$a \cdot A + b \cdot B \rightarrow P \qquad (2.1)$$

where a and b represent number of molecules, A and B the reactants, and P the product. The rate is expressed as $-d[A]/dt$, $-d[B]/dt$, and $d[P]/dt$, where t is the time and [A], [B], and [P] represent concentrations. The minus sign indicates a decrease in concentration. The rate has units of concentration divided by time (i.e., $M\ s^{-1}$, $M\ h^{-1}$, or $mg\ ml^{-1}\ h^{-1}$). The order of reaction is the sum of a and b (i.e., the number of molecules participating in the reaction). For example, hydrolysis of methyl salicylate in aqueous solution follows the chemical equation:

$$(2.2)$$

where methyl salicylate and water are the reactants and salicylic acid and methanol the products. The reaction is first order with respect to methyl salicylate and first order with respect to water, but overall the reaction is second order. A reaction involving only one reactant molecule is called *unimolecular*; a reaction involving two molecules is called *bimolecular*; and a reaction involving three molecules is called *termolecular*. Radioactive decay, in which particles are emitted from an atom, is an example of a unimolecular reaction. Bimolecular reactions, in which two molecules react to form product(s), are very common chemical reactions. Ester hydrolysis, shown in Eq. 2.2, is an example of bimolecular reaction. Termolecular reactions, in which three molecules collide simultaneously to react, are rare.

2.1 ZERO-ORDER REACTIONS

A zero-order reaction is a reaction in which rate is independent of the reactant concentration:

$$-\frac{d[A]}{dt} = k_0 \qquad (2.3)$$

where k_0 is the rate constant for the zero-order reaction. Although "pure" zero-order reactions are rather uncommon, *apparent* (or *pseudo*) zero-order reactions are frequently observed in pharmaceutical products, such as drug suspensions. Under these conditions, the drug degradation follows first-order kinetics, but the solid drug present in the suspension dissolves and maintains the concentration of dissolved drug ([A]) constant:

$$-\frac{d[A]}{dt} = k_1[A] = k_0 \qquad (2.4)$$

where k_1 is the first-order rate constant and [A] is the concentration of dissolved drug. Rearrangement of Eq. 2.3 gives Eq. 2.5:

$$[A] = [A]_0 - k_0 t \qquad (2.5)$$

where $[A]_0$ is the total drug concentration at time zero. The rate constant is obtained by plotting the change in [A] over time (Fig. 2.1).

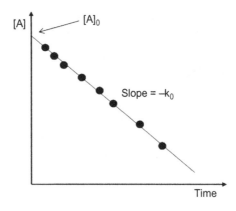

Figure 2.1 Zero-order plot of [A] versus time. [A]$_0$ is the y-intercept.

The *half-life* ($t_{1/2}$) of the reaction is the time required for the total drug concentration to fall to half of its value as measured at the beginning of the time period (i.e., $[A]_0$ to $\frac{1}{2}[A]_0$), and the *shelf-life* (t_{90} or t_{95}) is the time required for the total drug concentration to fall to 90% or 95% of its initial value.

$$t_{1/2} = \frac{0.50[A]_0}{k_0} \tag{2.6}$$

$$t_{90} = \frac{0.10[A]_0}{k_0} \tag{2.7}$$

$$t_{95} = \frac{0.05[A]_0}{k_0} \tag{2.8}$$

Thus, both the half-life and the shelf-life of zero-order reactions depend on the initial drug concentration.

2.2 FIRST-ORDER REACTIONS

The rate of a first-order reaction is directly proportional to a single reactant concentration:

$$A \rightarrow P \tag{2.9}$$

$$-\frac{d[A]}{dt} = k_1[A] \tag{2.10}$$

where k_1 is the first-order rate constant and $[A]$ is the reactant (i.e., drug) concentration. The rate of drug disappearance is equal to the rate of product formation (Fig. 2.2):

$$-\frac{d[A]}{dt} = \frac{d[P]}{dt} = k_1[A] \tag{2.11}$$

where $[A] = [P]$ at $t_{1/2}$. Rearrangement of Eq. 2.10 and integration from $t = 0$ ($[A]_0$) to time t ($[A]$) gives:

$$-\frac{d[A]}{[A]} = k_1 dt \tag{2.12}$$

$$-\int_{[A]_0}^{[A]} \frac{d[A]}{[A]} = \int_0^t k_1 dt \tag{2.13}$$

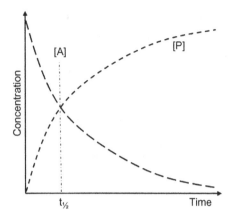

Figure 2.2 Plot of [A] and [P] versus time.

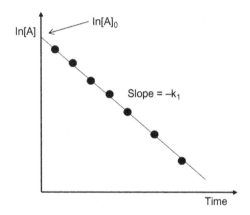

Figure 2.3 First-order plot of ln[A] versus time. ln[A]₀ is the y-intercept.

$$[A] = [A]_0 e^{-k_1 t} \qquad (2.14)$$

$$\ln[A] = \ln[A]_0 - k_1 t \qquad (2.15)$$

Eq. 2.15 describes a linear plot (Fig. 2.3).

Eq. 2.15 can also be written as:

$$\log[A] = \log[A]_0 - k_1 t/2.303 \qquad (2.16)$$

where $\ln[A] = 2.303\log[A]$. The common logarithm (log) is based on 10 (also called the decimal logarithm) and is generally used in older textbooks, as well as by some drug regulatory authorities, to describe drug degradation kinetics. However, in this book we mainly use the natural logarithm (ln) that is based on e ($=2.7183\ldots$) avoiding the conversion factor of 2.303.

For first-order reactions $t_{1/2}$, t_{90}, and t_{95} are independent of the initial drug concentration. For example, according to Eq. 2.15 $t_{1/2}$ (the time it takes $[A]_0$ to reach $\frac{1}{2}[A]_0$) can be calculated as follows:

$$\ln(\tfrac{1}{2}[A]_0) = \ln[A]_0 - k_1 t_{1/2} \tag{2.17}$$

Rearranging Eq. 2.17 gives:

$$t_{1/2} = \frac{\ln 2}{k_1} = \frac{0.693}{k_1} \tag{2.18}$$

Likewise, the following equations for t_{90} and t_{95} can be obtained:

$$t_{90} = \frac{0.105}{k_1} \tag{2.19}$$

$$t_{95} = \frac{0.0513}{k_1} \tag{2.20}$$

Example 2.1: Hydrolysis of homatropine in aqueous solution
Homatropine is an ester that undergoes hydrolysis in aqueous solutions [1]. Samples were collected and the homatropine concentration at various time points calculated:

Time (h)	[Homatropine] (M)	ln[Homatropine]
1.4	0.026	−3.650
3.0	0.024	−3.730
6.0	0.021	−3.863
9.0	0.018	−4.017
12	0.015	−4.200
17	0.012	−4.423

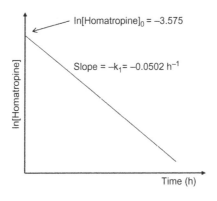

The following values can then be calculated from the graph:

The initial homatropine concentration $= e^{-3.575} = 0.028$ M

The first-order rate constant $= k_1 = 5.05 \times 10^{-2}\,h^{-1}$

$$\text{The half-life} = t_{1/2} = \frac{\ln 2}{k_1} = \frac{0.693}{5.05 \times 10^{-2}\,h^{-1}} = 13.7\,h$$

$$\text{The shelf-life} = t_{90} = \frac{0.105}{k_1} = \frac{0.105}{5.05 \times 10^{-2}\,h^{-1}} = 2.1\,h$$

Example 2.2: Hydrolysis of amoxicillin in aqueous drug suspension
Amoxicillin (MW 365.4 g/mol) is a β-lactam antibiotic that undergoes hydrolysis in aqueous solutions [2]. Due to its instability, aqueous amoxicillin mixtures are prepared in the pharmacy just before dispensing by suspending drug granules in purified water. At pH 6.0 and 25°C, the value of the first-order rate constant (k_1) is $1.26 \times 10^{-3}\,h^{-1}$. Under these conditions, the solubility of amoxicillin is 3.4 mg/ml ($= 3.4$ g/l). What is the shelf-life (t_{90}) of an amoxicillin mixture that contains 50 mg/ml of amoxicillin in an aqueous suspension?

Answer:

In a suspension, the amoxicillin degradation follows apparent zero-order kinetics (Eq. 2.4) in which [Amox] is constant and equal to the amoxicillin solubility 3.4 mg/ml. The zero-order rate constant is calculated as follows:

$$-\frac{d[\text{Amox}]}{dt} = k_1[\text{Amox}] = k_0 = 1.26 \times 10^{-3}h^{-1}\,\frac{3.4\,\text{g/l}}{365.4\,\text{g/mol}}$$

$$= 1.17 \times 10^{-5}\,\frac{\text{mol}}{\text{liter}\cdot h}$$

The initial amoxicillin concentration in the suspension:

$$[\text{A}]_0 = \frac{50\,\text{g/l}}{365.4\,\text{g/mol}} = 0.1368\,\text{mol/l}$$

The solid amoxicillin in the suspension is essentially stable in comparison to dissolved amoxicillin and, thus, amoxicillin degradation in the solid state can be ignored. t_{90} is defined as the time for the original potency of the active drug to be reduced to 90% (i.e., from 0.1368 to 0.1232 mol/liter) (Eq. 2.7):

$$t_{90} = \frac{0.10\,[\text{A}]_0}{k_0} = \frac{0.10 \cdot 0.1368\,\text{mol/liter}}{1.17 \times 10^{-5}\,\frac{\text{mol}}{\text{liter}\cdot h}} = 1169\,h = 49\,\text{days}$$

If all amoxicillin is in solution, then t_{90} will be independent of $[Amox]_0$ (Eq. 2.19):

$$t_{90} = \frac{0.105}{k_1} = \frac{0.105}{1.26 \times 10^{-3} \text{ h}^{-1}} = 83 \text{ h} = 3.5 \text{ days}$$

Thus, formulating amoxicillin as an aqueous suspension instead of an aqueous solution increases t_{90} from 3.5 to 49 days. The expiration date after forming an amoxicillin mixture is frequently 14 days. Small changes in pH and temperature can have significant affect on the shelf-life. For example, an increase in pH from 6.0 to 7.0 can result in a 10 fold decrease in the shelf-life, or from 49 days to 4.9 days. The shelf-life will increase if we lower the temperature from room temperature (about 25°C) to refrigerator termperature (about 5°C). Thus, due to variable storage conditions, the expiration date is often much shorter than the shelf-life at a given storage condition.

The half-life of amoxicillin in the mixture at pH 6.0 and 25°C is (Eq. 2.6):

$$t_{1/2} = \frac{0.50[Amox]_0}{k_0} = \frac{0.50 \cdot 0.1368 \text{ mol/liter}}{1.17 \times 10^{-5} \frac{\text{mol}}{\text{liter·h}}} = 5.8 \times 10^3 \text{ h} = 240 \text{ days}$$

Example 2.3: Calculation of a first-order rate constant from peak heights
Since rates of first-order drug degradations are independent of the actual drug concentration in the reaction media, the actual drug concentration does not need to be known for the calculation of constants. For example, an anticancer drug was dissolved in pure water at 80°C and the amount of drug in the aqueous solution determined at various time points by injecting samples into HPLC is:

Time (min)	Peak Height (cm)
10	13.87
20	11.59
30	9.58
40	8.00
60	5.53
80	3.78

Calculate the observed rate constant (k_{obs}) and the shelf-life (t_{90}).

Answer:

The peak height (PH) is proportional to the actual drug concentration in the aqueous solution or $(PH) \times constant = [A]$. Substitution into Eq. 2.15 gives:

$$\ln((PH) \times constant) = \ln((PH)_0 \times constant) - k_1 t \text{ or}$$

$$\ln(PH) + \ln(constant) = \ln(PH)_0 + \ln(constant) - k_1 t$$

Deleting ln(constant) gives

$$\ln(PH) = \ln(PH)_0 - k_1 t$$

Plotting this equation gives:

Time (min)	PH (cm)	ln(PH)
10	13.87	2.63
20	11.59	2.45
30	9.58	2.26
40	8.00	2.08
60	5.53	1.71
80	3.78	1.33

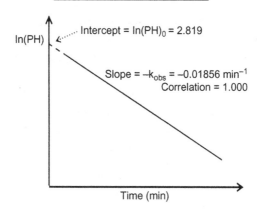

$$k_{obs} = 1.86 \cdot 10^{-2} \text{ min}^{-1} \qquad t_{90} = \frac{0.105}{k_{obs}} = 5.7 \text{ min}$$

2.3 SECOND-ORDER REACTIONS

The rate of a second-order reaction is proportional to the concentration of two reactants:

$$A + B \rightarrow P \tag{2.21}$$

$$-\frac{d[A]}{dt} = -\frac{d[B]}{dt} = k_2[A][B] \tag{2.22}$$

where k_2 is the second-order rate constant and [A] and [B] are the reactant concentrations.

$$-\int_{[A]_0}^{[A]} \frac{d[A]}{[A][B]} = \int_0^t k_2 dt \tag{2.23}$$

Integration of Eq. 2.23 gives:

$$\frac{1}{[A]_0 - [B]_0} \cdot \left[\ln \frac{[B]_0[A]}{[A]_0[B]} \right] = k_2 t \tag{2.24}$$

Eq. 2.24 can be rearranged to:

$$\frac{1}{t([A]_0 - [B]_0)} \cdot \left[\ln \frac{[B]_0[A]}{[A]_0[B]} \right] = k_2 \tag{2.25}$$

A simpler form of second-order reaction is obtained if [A] = [B] or if two molecules of A react:

$$-\frac{d[A]}{dt} = k_2[A]^2 \tag{2.26}$$

$$-\frac{d[A]}{[A]^2} = k_2 dt \tag{2.27}$$

$$-\int_{[A]_0}^{[A]} \frac{d[A]}{[A]^2} = \int_0^t k_2 dt \tag{2.28}$$

$$\frac{1}{[A]} - \frac{1}{[A]_0} = k_2 t \tag{2.29}$$

$$t = \frac{1}{k_2} \left(\frac{1}{[A]} - \frac{1}{[A]_0} \right) \tag{2.30}$$

According to 2.30 the half-life is:

$$t_{1/2} = \frac{1}{k_2[A]_0}$$

(2.31)

Example 2.4: Hydrolysis of an ester under alkaline conditions

Ethyl acetate undergoes hydrolysis in aqueous alkaline solutions containing equal concentrations of both the ester and sodium hydroxide or 0.020 M [3]. Samples were collected and the ethyl acetate concentration was determined at two time points:

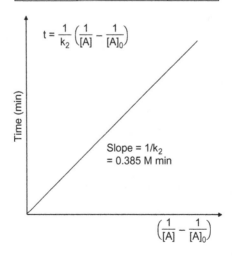

The initial concentrations of both reactants are the same and, thus, Eq. 2.30 can be used to calculate the second-order rate constant.

Time (min)	[ethyl acetate] (M)	$\frac{1}{[A]} - \frac{1}{[A]_0}$
0	0.020	–
20	0.011	40.91
40	0.007	92.86

$$\frac{1}{k_2} = 0.385 \text{ M min} \Rightarrow k_2 = 2.60 \text{ M}^{-1} \text{ min}^{-1}$$

Since the initial concentrations of both the ester and the sodium hydroxide are identical, Eq. 2.31 can be used to calculate the half-life:

$$t_{1/2} = \frac{1}{k_2[A]_0} = \frac{1}{2.60 \text{ M}^{-1} \text{ min}^{-1} \cdot 0.020 \text{ M}} \approx 19.2 \text{ min}$$

2.4 THIRD-ORDER REACTIONS

An example of a third-order reaction is the acid catalyzed hydrolysis of an ester:

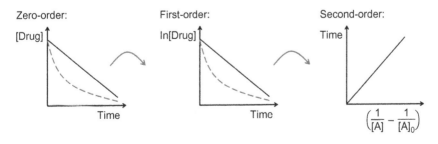

$$-\frac{d[\text{Ester}]}{dt} = k_3[\text{Ester}][\text{H}^+][\text{H}_2\text{O}] \qquad (2.32)$$

However, since in aqueous solutions the water concentration is essentially constant ($[\text{H}_2\text{O}] = 55.55$ M), the product of k_3 and $[\text{H}_2\text{O}]$ is also constant and equal to k_2 (i.e., the second-order rate constant):

$$-\frac{d[\text{Ester}]}{dt} = k_3[\text{Ester}][\text{H}^+][\text{H}_2\text{O}] = k_2[\text{Ester}][\text{H}^+] \qquad (2.33)$$

Here k_2 is the apparent (or pseudo) second-order rate constant for the ester hydrolysis.

2.5 DETERMINATION OF THE ORDER OF A REACTION

The best way to determine the order of a reaction is to plot the data according to the equation for zero-order (Eq. 2.5), first-order (Eq. 2.15), or second-order (Eq. 2.30) reactions:

If a linear zero-order plot is obtained, then the reaction follows zero-order kinetics. If a nonlinear plot is observed, then replot the data according to a first-order equation. If a linear plot is observed, then the reaction is first-order; if not, then try a second-order plot, and so on.

The half-life method can also be used to determine the order of a reaction. From Eqs. 2.6, 2.18, and 2.31 it can be seen that:

$$t_{1/2} \propto \frac{1}{([A]_0)^{n-1}} \quad n \neq 1 \tag{2.34}$$

where $[A]_0$ is the initial reactant (drug) concentration and n is the reaction order. Eq. 2.35 and 2.36 are based on Eq. 2.34. In Eq. 2.35, $t_{1/2}$ is determined at two different $[A]_0$ values:

$$n = \frac{\log\left(\frac{t_{1/2}^1}{t_{1/2}^2}\right)}{\log\left(\frac{[A]_0^2}{[A]_0^1}\right)} + 1 \tag{2.35}$$

In Eq. 2.36, $t_{1/2}$ is determined at several different $[A]_0$ values and n is determined from a linear plot of the results (Fig. 2.4):

$$\log t_{1/2} = \log\left[\frac{2^{n-1} - 1}{k(n-1)}\right] + (1 - n)\log[A]_0 \tag{2.36}$$

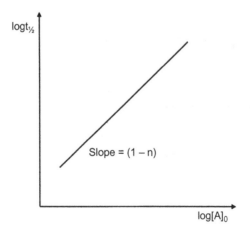

Figure 2.4 Half-life plot for reaction order determination.

2.6 COMPLEX REACTIONS

Frequently, drug degradation does not follow a simple zero-, first-, or second-order kinetics, but follows a reversible reaction mechanism, following two or more degradation pathways or degrading to form several consecutive products. Under such conditions, the reaction cannot be described by a simple one-term mathematical equation and, consequently, is known as a *complex reaction*. Each mechanism is a special case and, thus, no general method can be applied to solve complex reactions. However, examples from the three main categories of complex reactions (i.e., reversible, parallel, and consecutive reactions) will be presented.

2.6.1 Reversible Reactions

The simplest reversible reaction is one in which the reaction proceeds via first-order kinetics in both directions:

$$A \underset{k_r}{\overset{k_f}{\rightleftarrows}} B \tag{2.37}$$

$$-\frac{d[A]}{dt} = \frac{d[B]}{dt} = k_f[A] - k_r[B] \tag{2.38}$$

where k_f and k_r represent the first-order rate constants for the forward and the reverse reactions, respectively. Due to the two variables ([A] and [B]) as well as the variable t, it is not possible to integrate Eq. 2.38 directly. It can, however, be seen that:

At $t = 0$: $[A] = [A]_0 \neq 0$ and $[B] = [B]_0 = 0$
At $t = t$: $[A] = [A]$ and $[B] = [A]_0 - [A]$
At $t = \to \infty$: $[A] = [A]_{eq}$ and $[B] = [B]_{eq}$

Thus Eq. 2.38 can be rearranged:

$$-\frac{d[A]}{dt} = k_f[A] - k_r[B] = k_f[A] - k_r([A]_0 - [A]) = (k_f + k_r)[A] - k_r[A]_0 \tag{2.39}$$

Rearranging this equation and integration gives:

$$-\int_{[A]_0}^{[A]} \frac{d[A]}{(k_f + k_r)[A] - k_r[A]_0} = \int_0^t dt \tag{2.40}$$

$$\ln[(k_f + k_r) \cdot [A] - k_r[A]_0] - \ln[k_f[A]_0] = -(k_f + k_r) \cdot t \tag{2.41}$$

$$\frac{(k_f + k_r)[A] - k_r[A]_0}{k_f[A]_0} = e^{-(k_f + k_r) \cdot t} \tag{2.42}$$

$$[A] = \frac{[A]_0(k_r + k_f e^{-(k_f + k_r) \cdot t})}{(k_f + k_r)} \tag{2.43}$$

If k_f, k_r, and $[A]_0$ are known, then $[A]$ can be calculated for any time point after initiation of the reaction. At equilibrium (i.e., when $t \to \infty$) then:

$$-\frac{d[A]}{dt} = k_f[A]_{eq} - k_r[B]_{eq} \to 0 \tag{2.44}$$

$$k_f[A]_{eq} = k_r[B]_{eq} \tag{2.45}$$

At $t = \infty$

$$k_f[A]_{eq} = k_r[A]_0 - k_r[A]_{eq} \tag{2.46}$$

and

$$\frac{k_r}{k_f + k_r}[A]_0 = [A]_{eq} \tag{2.47}$$

$$\frac{k_f}{k_f + k_r}[A]_0 = [B]_{eq} = [A]_0 - [A]_{eq} \tag{2.48}$$

Rearrangement of Eq. 2.41 gives:

$$\ln\left[\frac{k_f[A]_0}{(k_f + k_r)[A] - k_r[A]_0}\right] = (k_f + k_r) \cdot t \tag{2.49}$$

Eqs. 2.47 and 2.49 give Eq. 2.50:

$$\ln\left[\frac{k_f[A]_0}{(k_f + k_r)([A] - [A]_{eq})}\right] = (k_f + k_r) \cdot t \tag{2.50}$$

Eqs. 2.48 and 2.50 give Eq. 2.51:

$$\ln\left[\frac{[A]_0 - [A]_{eq}}{[A] - [A]_{eq}}\right] = (k_f + k_r) \cdot t \tag{2.51}$$

Rearrangement of Eq. 2.51 gives:

$$t = \frac{1}{(k_f + k_r)} \ln \frac{[A]_0 - [A]_{eq}}{[A] - [A]_{eq}}$$ (2.52)

From Eq. 2.45 it can be seen that:

$$K = \frac{[B]_{eq}}{[A]_{eq}} = \frac{k_f}{k_r}$$ (2.53)

where K is the equilibrium constant for the equation. Eqs. 2.52 and 2.53 describe a simple first-order equilibrium that is commonly observed during drug racemization when A and B are mirror images of each other. Under such conditions, K is equal to unity ($k_f = k_r \Rightarrow K = 1$). However, when A and B are not mirror images (e.g., epimerization), then k_f and k_r are not equal and, consequently, K is not equal to unity.

Eqs. 2.54 and 2.55 describe an equilibrium reaction in which the forward reaction is second-order and the reverse reaction is first-order:

$$A + B \underset{k_r}{\overset{k_f}{\rightleftharpoons}} C$$ (2.54)

$$-\frac{d[A]}{dt} = k_f[A][B] - k_r[C]$$ (2.55)

Second-order reversible reactions are more complicated to solve and, thus, second-order reactions are frequently run under apparent first-order conditions in which, for example, the concentration of B in Eq. 2.54 is fixed ([B] = constant).

Example 2.5: Epimerization of tetracycline
Tetracyclines have several asymmetric carbon atoms. In aqueous solutions, tetracyclines can undergo reversible isomerization in which the three-dimensional structure of one of the asymmetric carbons is changed to form 4-*epi*-tetracycline. *Epi*-tetracyclines have less antibacterial activity than the corresponding tetracyclines.

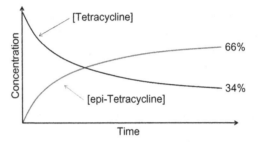

Tetracycline   4-*epi*-Tetracycline

The degradation of tetracycline in aqueous solution at elevated temperature was monitored and the concentrations of both tetracycline and *epi*-tetracycline were determined [4]:

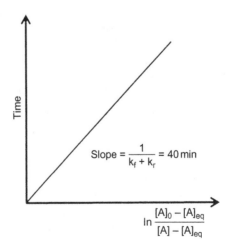

Notice that at equilibrium, tetracycline is 34% of the initial concentration and *epi*-tetracycline is 68%. The results were then plotted according to Eq. 2.52:

From the slope it can be calculated that $k_f + k_r = 2.50 \times 10^{-2}\,min^{-1}$. From the equilibrium concentrations and Eq. 2.53, it can be calculated that:

$$K = \frac{[epi\text{-}Tet]_{eq}}{[Tet]_{eq}} = \frac{66}{34} = 1.941 = \frac{k_f}{k_f} \tag{2.56}$$

$$k_f = 1.941 \times k_r \tag{2.57}$$

$$k_f + k_r = 2.50 \times 10^{-2}\,min^{-1} \tag{2.58}$$

Combining Eqs. 2.57 and 2.58 gives:

$$k_r = 8.50 \times 10^{-3}\,min^{-1} \text{ and } k_f = 1.65 \times 10^{-2}\,min^{-1}$$

2.6.2 Parallel Reactions

Sometimes, drug degradations follow two or more pathways. For two parallel reactions:

$$X \overset{k_A}{\underset{k_B}{\diagdown}} \begin{array}{l} A \\ B \end{array} \tag{2.59}$$

$$-\frac{d[X]}{dt} = \frac{d[A]}{dt} + \frac{d[B]}{dt} = k_A[X] + k_B[X] = (k_A + k_B)[X] = k_{exp}[X] \tag{2.60}$$

The experimental rate constant for the disappearance of X is k_{exp}. The relative values of k_A and k_B are determined by the relative amount of A and B formed during the degradation:

$$k_A = k_{exp}\frac{[A]}{[A] + [B]} \tag{2.61}$$

$$k_B = k_{exp}\frac{[B]}{[A] + [B]} \tag{2.62}$$

For three parallel reactions, the following equations are obtained:

$$X \overset{k_A}{\underset{k_C}{\longrightarrow}} \begin{array}{l} A \\ B \\ C \end{array} \tag{2.63}$$

$$-\frac{d[X]}{dt} = k_A[X] + k_B[X] + k_C[X] = (k_A + k_B + k_C)[X] = k_{exp}[X] \tag{2.64}$$

$$k_A = k_{exp}\frac{[A]}{[A] + [B] + [C]} \tag{2.65}$$

and so on. The ratio of the individual rate constants determines the ratio of the products formed: $k_A:k_B:k_C = [A]:[B]:[C]$.

Example 2.6: Degradation of pilocarpine

In aqueous solutions pilocarpine undergoes simultaneous epimerization and hydrolysis in which the initial degradation pathways are [5,6]:

where pilocarpine acid and *epi*-pilocarpine are being formed. At pH 10 and 25°C, the following rate constant was obtained when the concentration of pilocarpine was followed over time:

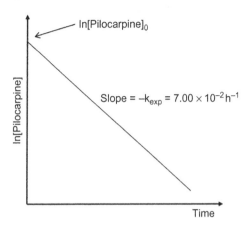

$$-\frac{d[\text{Pilocarpine}]}{dt} = k_A[\text{Pilocarpine}] + k_B[\text{Pilocarpine}] = k_{exp}[\text{Pilocarpine}]$$

$$= 7.00 \times 10^{-2} \ h^{-1}[\text{Pilocarpine}]$$

Analysis of the degradation products showed that the pilocarpine acid:*epi*-pilocarpine molar ratio was 8:2 or, in other words, that the acid was 80% of the product and the epimer was 20%:

$$\frac{[\text{Pilocarpine acid}]}{[\text{Pilocarpine acid}] + [epi\text{-Pilocarpine}]} = 0.80$$

$$k_H = k_{exp} \cdot 0.80 = 7.00 \times 10^{-2} \cdot 0.80 = 5.6 \times 10^{-2} \ h^{-1}$$

$$k_E = k_{exp} \cdot 0.20 = 7.00 \times 10^{-2} \cdot 0.20 = 1.4 \times 10^{-2} \ h^{-1}$$

2.6.3 Consecutive Reactions

Consecutive reactions, in which an intermediate is formed and then degraded, are fairly common in organic chemistry. The simplest form of consecutive reactions consists of two first-order consecutive reactions:

$$A \xrightarrow{k_A} B \xrightarrow{k_B} C \tag{2.66}$$

$$-\frac{d[A]}{dt} = k_A[A] \qquad\qquad (2.10)$$

$$\frac{d[B]}{dt} = k_A[A] - k_B[B] \qquad\qquad (2.67)$$

$$\frac{d[C]}{dt} = k_B[B] \qquad\qquad (2.68)$$

Integration of Eq. 2.10 gives:

$$[A] = [A]_0 e^{-k_A t} \qquad\qquad (2.14)$$

Combining Eqs. 2.67 and 2.14 gives:

$$\frac{d[B]}{dt} = k_A[A]_0 e^{-k_A t} - k_B[B] \qquad\qquad (2.69)$$

Integration of Eq. 2.69 gives:

$$[B] = \frac{k_A[A]_0}{(k_B - k_A)} (e^{-k_A t} - e^{-k_B t}) \qquad\qquad (2.70)$$

Furthermore, it can be seen that:

$$[A]_0 = [A] + [B] + [C] \qquad\qquad (2.71)$$

Example 2.7: Degradation of an aspirin prodrug
Prodrugs are inactive molecules that are metabolized to the active drug in vivo. Many prodrugs are chemically unstable in aqueous solutions. The following is an example of such a prodrug, (A), that hydrolyzes in aqueous solutions to form aspirin (B) that is hydrolyzed further to form salicylic acid [7]:

(A)   (B)   (C)

At pH 8.0 and 51°C, almost all of the prodrug (>94%) is hydrolyzed according to this mechanism, and under this condition the rate constants have the following values:

$$k_A = 6.10 \times 10^{-2} \text{ min}^{-1}$$
$$k_B = 2.14 \times 10^{-3} \text{ min}^{-1}$$

The half-life of the prodrug is:

$$t_{1/2} = \frac{0.693}{6.10 \times 10^{-2}} = 11.36 \text{ min} \approx 11 \text{ min}$$

The concentrations (in %) of A, B, and C at t = 11 min are calculated as follows:

$$[A] = [A]_0 e^{-k_A t} = 100 \times e^{-6.10 \times 10^{-2} \times 11} = 100 \times 0.51 = 51\%$$

$$[B] = \frac{6.10 \times 10^{-2} \times 100}{(2.14 \times 10^{-3} - 6.10 \times 10^{-2})} (e^{-6.10 \times 10^{-2} \times 11} - e^{-2.14 \times 10^{-3} \times 11})$$
$$= -103.64 \times (0.5111 - 0.9767) = 48\%$$

$$[C] = [A]_0 - [A] - [B] = 100 - 51 - 48 = 1\%$$

More exact calculations will show that [C] at 11 minutes is close to 0.5%. For this aspirin prodrug under these conditions, $k_A \approx 30 \cdot k_B$ and, thus, there will be considerable buildup of B in the solution. The concentration-time profile could look something like this:

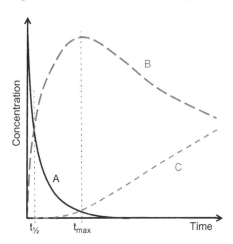

$$t_{max} = \frac{\ln(k_A/k_B)}{k_A - k_B} = \frac{\ln(6.10 \times 10^{-2}/2.14 \times 10^{-3})}{6.10 \times 10^{-2} - 2.14 \times 10^{-3}} = 56.7 \, \text{min} \quad (2.72)$$

$$[B]_{max} = [A]_0 \left(\frac{k_A}{k_B}\right)^{\frac{k_B}{k_A - k_B}} = 100 \left(\frac{6.10 \times 10^{-2}}{2.14 \times 10^{-3}}\right)^{\frac{2.14 \times 10^{-3}}{6.10 \times 10^{-2} - 2.14 \times 10^{-3}}}$$

$$= 100 \times 28.5^{0.0364} \approx 100\% \quad (2.73)$$

2.6.4 Steady-State Approximation

In Example 2.4, there was a considerable buildup of the intermediate B before it slowly degraded to form C. In other instances, the concentration of a very reactive intermediate remains low during the course of the reaction. In such cases, steady-state approximation can be applied to simplify complex mathematical rate expressions. An example of such a reaction is the degradation of diazepam in aqueous acidic solutions (Fig. 2.5) [8].

In the first reaction, the 1,4-benzodiazepine ring of drug is opened to form an amide (B) that then is hydrolyzed to form 2-(N-methylamino)-5-chlorobenzophenone (C) and glycine (D). Intermediate C is reactive and consequently is present only at very low concentrations or, in other words, it degrades soon after it has formed. Furthermore, the first degradation step is a reversible reaction making exact integration of the rate equations involved very difficult. The following is a steady-state approximation of the rate equations:

$$A \underset{k_{-1}}{\overset{k_1}{\rightleftharpoons}} B \xrightarrow{k_2} C \quad (2.74)$$

$$-\frac{d[A]}{dt} = k_1[A] - k_{-1}[B] \quad (2.75)$$

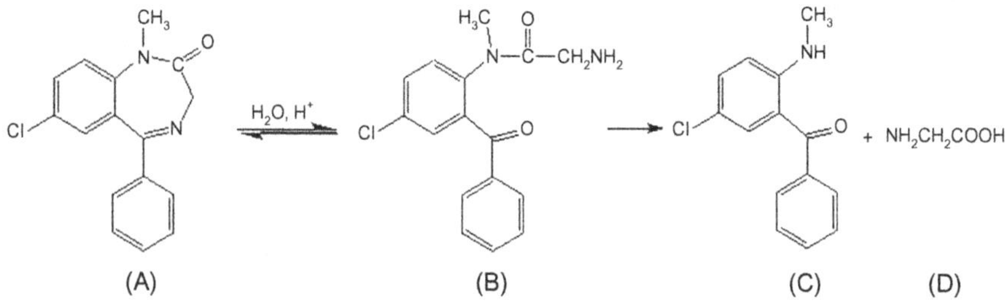

Figure 2.5 Degradation of diazepam (A) in aqueous acidic solution.

$$\frac{d[B]}{dt} = k_1[A] - k_{-1}[B] - k_2[B] \qquad (2.76)$$

$$\frac{d[C]}{dt} = k_2[B] \qquad (2.77)$$

If we assume that [B] is constant during the course of the reaction (expressed by $[B]_{ss}$), then Eq. 2.76 becomes:

$$\frac{d[B]_{ss}}{dt} = k_1[A] - k_{-1}[B]_{ss} - k_2[B]_{ss} = 0 \qquad (2.78)$$

Rearrangement of Eq. 2.78 gives:

$$[B]_{ss} = \frac{k_1[A]}{k_{-1} + k_2} \qquad (2.79)$$

$$-\frac{d[A]}{dt} = k_1[A] - k_{-1}[B] = k_1[A] - k_{-1}\frac{k_1[A]}{k_{-1} + k_2} \qquad (2.80)$$

Rearrangement of Eq. 2.80 gives:

$$-\frac{d[A]}{dt} = \frac{k_1 k_2}{k_{-1} + k_2}[A] = k'[A] \qquad (2.81)$$

Thus, a complex consecutive reaction mechanism has been converted to a simple first-order reaction that can be described by Eqs. 2.14 and 2.15.

2.6.5 Michaelis–Menten Equation

One of the best known and simplest models used to describe enzyme kinetics is when one enzyme (E) molecule combines with one substrate (S) molecule to form a complex (ES) that breaks down to form the product P:

$$E + S \underset{k_2}{\overset{k_1}{\rightleftharpoons}} ES \xrightarrow{k_3} P \qquad (2.82)$$

A steady-state approximation is used to solve the rate equations:

$$-\frac{d[S]}{dt} = k_1[E][S] - k_2[ES] \qquad (2.83)$$

$$\frac{d[ES]}{dt} = k_1[E][S] - k_2[ES] - k_3[ES] \qquad (2.84)$$

$$\frac{d[P]}{dt} = k_3[ES] \tag{2.85}$$

If we assume that [ES] remains essentially constant during the course of the reaction (expressed by $[ES]_{ss}$), then Eq. 2.84 becomes:

$$\frac{d[ES]_{ss}}{dt} = k_1[E][S] - k_2[ES]_{ss} - k_3[ES]_{ss} = 0 \tag{2.86}$$

Rearrangement of Eq. 2.86 gives:

$$[ES]_{ss} = \frac{k_1[E][S]}{k_2 + k_3} \tag{2.87}$$

The total enzyme concentration ($[E]_T$) is the sum of the free (unbound) enzyme concentration ([E]) and the concentration of the enzyme-substrate complex ([ES]), or at steady-state:

$$[E]_T = [E] + [ES]_{ss} \tag{2.88}$$

Combining Eqs. 2.87 and 2.88 gives:

$$[ES]_{ss} = \frac{k_1[E][S]}{k_2 + k_3} = \frac{k_1[E]_T[S] - k_1[ES]_{ss}[S]}{k_2 + k_3} \tag{2.89}$$

Rearrangement of Eq. 2.89 gives:

$$[ES]_{ss} = \frac{k_1[E]_T[S]}{(k_2 + k_3) + k_1[S]} \tag{2.90}$$

The Michaelis−Menten constant (K_m) is defined as:

$$K_m = \frac{k_2 + k_3}{k_1} \tag{2.91}$$

Combining Eqs. 2.90 and 2.91 gives:

$$[ES]_{ss} = \frac{[E]_T[S]}{K_m + [S]} \tag{2.92}$$

Combining Eqs. 2.85 and 2.92 gives the Michaelis−Menten equation:

$$\frac{d[P]}{dt} = V = k_3 \frac{[E]_T[S]}{K_m + [S]} \tag{2.93}$$

where V is the velocity (d[P]/dt). Maximum velocity (V_{max}) is obtained when the enzyme is saturated with the substrate (i.e., when $[ES]_{ss}$ in Eq. 2.85 is equal to $[E]_T$) and, thus, V_{max} is defined as:

$$V_{max} = k_3[E]_T \qquad (2.94)$$

Combining Eqs. 2.93 and 2.94 gives the common form of the Michaelis–Menten equation:

$$V = \frac{V_{max}[S]}{K_m + [S]} \qquad (2.95)$$

At steady state, the substrate disappears at the same rate the product appears (i.e., $-d[S]/dt = d[P]/dt$) and thus:

$$-\frac{d[S]}{dt} = \frac{V_{max}[S]}{K_m + [S]} \qquad (2.96)$$

This equation can then be rearranged to obtain the values of V_{max} and K_m.

Example 2.8: Enzyme catalyzed drug degradation
Enzyme catalyzed drug degradation was measured in vitro by monitoring the drug concentration through time. Calculate V_{max} and K_M from the values given in the table below.

t (min)	[S] (μg/ml)
0	55.00
40	38.02
70	25.51
150	2.38
165	0.93

First, we need to rearrange Eq. 2.96:

$$-\frac{d[S]}{[S]}(K_m + [S]) = V_{max}\, dt \qquad (2.97)$$

Integration of Eq. 2.97 gives:

$$\frac{[S]_0 - [S]_t}{t} = V_{max} - \frac{K_m}{t}\ln\frac{[S]_0}{[S]_t} \qquad (2.98)$$

Thus, plotting $\frac{[S]_0 - [S]_t}{t}$ *versus* $\frac{\ln\frac{[S]_0}{[S]_t}}{t}$ will give a linear plot:

Time (min)	$[S]_0 - [S]_t$ (μg/ml)	t (min)	$\frac{[S]_0 - [S]_t}{t}$ (μg/ml/min)	$\ln\frac{[S]_0}{[S]_t}$	$\frac{\ln\frac{[S]_0}{[S]_t}}{t}$ (min^{-1})
0–40	16.98	40	0.4245	0.3692	0.00923
40–70	29.49	70	0.4213	0.7683	0.01098
70–150	52.62	150	0.3508	3.1402	0.02093
150–165	54.07	165	0.3277	4.0799	0.02477

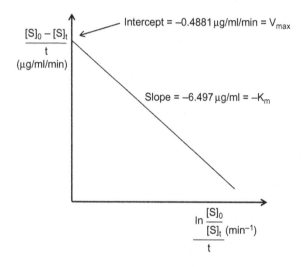

Here $V_{max} = 0.49\ \mu g\ ml^{-1}\ min^{-1}$ and $K_m = 6.50\ \mu g/ml$.

At very low substrate concentration when $[S] \ll K_m$, Eq. 2.96 approaches a first-order reaction:

$$-\frac{d[S]}{dt} = \frac{V_{max}[S]}{K_m + [S]} \approx \frac{V_{max}[S]}{K_m} = k'[S] \qquad (2.99)$$

where k' is the observed first-order rate constant. In the example above k' is:

$$k' = \frac{0.49}{6.50} = 7.5 \times 10^{-2}\ min^{-1}$$

2.6.6 Rate-Limiting Step

In most cases, drug degradation proceeds through several steps in which one step is much slower than the subsequent steps, leading to the

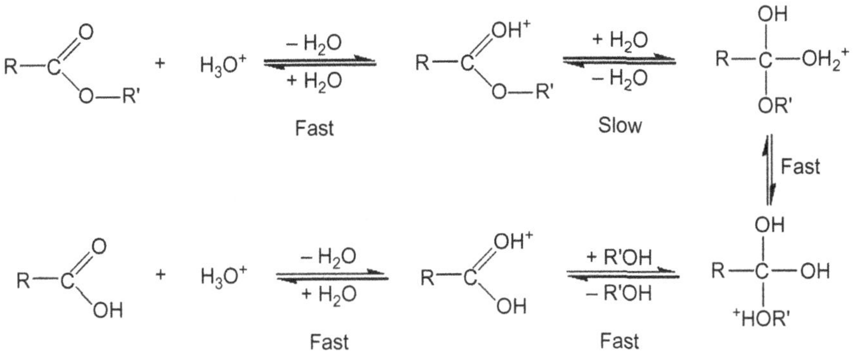

Figure 2.6 Specific acid-catalyzed ester hydrolysis in aqueous solution.

degradation product. For example, in specific acid-catalyzed ester hydrolysis, the nucleophilic attack of water to form the tetrahedral is the slowest step, while the subsequent steps are much faster (Fig. 2.6).

The rate at which the ester is hydrolyzed depends on the rates of all of the steps preceding the slow step, but not on any of the following steps and, thus, ester hydrolysis in aqueous acidic solution can be expressed as:

$$-\frac{d[\text{Ester}]}{dt} = k_H[\text{Ester}]\left[H_3O^+\right]$$

where k_H is the second-order rate constant for the ester hydrolysis under acidic conditions and $[H_3O^+]$ is the proton concentration that is most often expressed as $[H^+]$. The slow nucleophilic attack of water to form the tetrahedral is the rate-limiting step (sometimes called rate-determining step).

2.7 EFFECT OF TEMPERATURE

According to the *collision theory*, molecules must collide for a chemical reaction to occur, but only a portion of the colliding molecules have sufficient energy and orientation for a reaction to proceed and form products. The minimum amount of energy needed for a reaction to proceed is called energy of activation (E_a). The average kinetic energy of the molecules increases with increasing temperature. As the temperature increases, a higher fraction of molecules will have sufficient

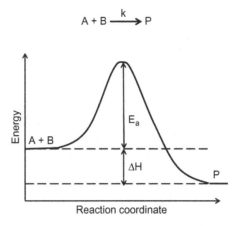

Figure 2.7 The energy required for two molecules (A and B) to react to form a product (P).

energy to overcome the activation energy barrier (Fig. 2.7). Thus, the reaction rate constant (k) increases and the reaction proceeds faster with increasing temperature.

According to the Collision theory:

$$k = PZe^{-\frac{E_a}{RT}} \tag{2.100}$$

where P is the probability factor (sometimes called stearic factor) indicating how critical molecular orientation is during the collision, Z is the collision frequency (i.e., number of collisions per unit time), R is the gas constant, and T is the absolute temperature. The value of P is usually between 1 (the molecular orientation is not critical) and 10^{-9} (the molecular orientation is very critical). The fraction of collisions of sufficient energy to give a product is $e^{-\frac{E_a}{RT}}$. Eq. 2.100 can also be written as:

$$k = Ae^{-\frac{E_a}{RT}} \tag{2.101}$$

where A is the frequency factor. Eq. 2.101 is called the *Arrhenius equation* and is commonly used to explain how temperature affects the chemical stability of drugs in solutions and even in the solid state. The natural logarithm of Eq. 2.101 gives an equation of a straight line (Fig. 2.8):

$$\ln k = \ln A - \frac{E_a}{R \cdot T} \tag{2.102}$$

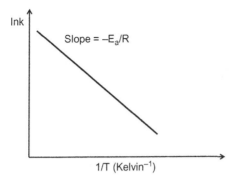

Figure 2.8 Arrhenius plot used to determine E_a and to extrapolate reaction rates determined at elevated temperatures to, for example, room temperature.

where E_a can be calculated from the slope. The value of E_a is frequently between 50 and 100 kJ/mol (between 12 and 24 kcal/mol) indicating that the value of k doubles to triples for every $10°C$ temperature increase. For a given reaction under a given reaction condition (i.e., reaction media, pH, etc.), the following equations can be used to calculate k-values at different temperatures:

$$\ln\frac{k_2}{k_1} = -\frac{E_a}{R}\left[\frac{1}{T_2} - \frac{1}{T_1}\right] \tag{2.103}$$

$$\ln\frac{k_2}{k_1} = -\frac{E_a(T_2 - T_1)}{RT_1T_2} \tag{2.104}$$

Thus, if E_a is known and the rate constant (k_1) at a given temperature is T_1, then it is possible to calculate k_2 at temperature T_2 using either Eq. 2.103 or 2.104.

Example 2.9: Calculation of E_a, $t_{½}$, and t_{90}
Atropine is an ester that is hydrolyzed in aqueous solutions [9,10]. The following data for atropine hydrolysis was obtained for an aqueous atropine solution:

Temperature (°C)	k (min⁻¹)
60	$8.45\ 10^{-6}$
50	$3.94\ 10^{-6}$
40	$1.77\ 10^{-6}$

Using the data in the table, calculate A, E_a, $t_{1/2}$, and t_{90} at room temperature (25°C).

We start by plotting the data according to Eq. 2.102.

$$\ln k = \ln A - \frac{E_a}{R}\cdot\frac{1}{T}$$

Then we need to convert the data from the table to the Y (lnk) and X (1/T) values:

Temperature (°C)	Temperature (K)	1/T (K⁻¹)	k (min⁻¹)	lnk
60	333.15	$3.002\ 10^{-3}$	$8.45\ 10^{-6}$	-11.681
50	323.15	$3,095\ 10^{-3}$	$3.94\ 10^{-6}$	-12.444
40	313.15	$3.193\ 10^{-3}$	$1.77\ 10^{-6}$	-13.245

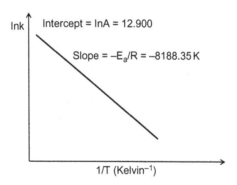

$R = 8.3143\ J\ mol^{-1}\ K^{-1} = 1.9872\ cal^{-1}\ mol^{-1}\ K^{-1}$
$E_a = Slope \times R$ or
$E_a = 68.08\ kJ/mol = 16.27\ kcal/mol$
$A = e^{Intercept} = 4.00 \cdot 10^5\ min^{-1}$

According to the definition, values of both A and E_a are independent of temperature but depend on reaction and media conditions such as pH.

At 25°C (298 K) the values are:

$A = 4.00 \cdot 10^5 \text{ min}^{-1}$

$E_a = 68.08 \text{ kJ/mol}$

From Eq. 2.101: $k = 4.00 \cdot 10^5 \times e^{-\frac{68080}{8.3143 \cdot 298}} = 4.66 \cdot 10^{-7} \text{min}^{-1}$

From Eq. 2.18: $t_{1/2} = \frac{\ln 2}{k_1} = \frac{0.693}{4.66 \cdot 10^{-7}} = 1.487 \cdot 10^6 \text{ min} = 2.8 \text{ years}$

From Eq. 2.19: $t_{90} = \frac{0.105}{k_1} = \frac{0.105}{4.66 \cdot 10^{-7}} = 2.25 \cdot 10^5 \text{ min} = 156 \text{ days}$

2.7.1 Q_{10} Values and Shelf-Life Estimation

Q_{10} factors were introduced for quick estimation of shelf-life when drugs are stored under different storage temperatures (e.g., room temperature (25°C), cold room (15°C), and refrigerator (5°C)) [11]. The Q_{10} factor is defined as the rate constant increase when the temperature is increased by 10 K (or 10°C):

$$Q_{10} = \frac{k_{(T+10)}}{k_T} \tag{2.105}$$

$$Q_{10} = \frac{k_{(T+10)}}{k_T} = e^{-\frac{E_a}{R} \cdot \left(\frac{1}{T+10} - \frac{1}{T}\right)} \tag{2.106}$$

The value of Q_{10} is proportional to E_a, meaning that Q_{10} increases with increasing E_a but is inversely proportional to the temperature, decreasing with increasing temperature as shown in the table below:

E_a (kJ/mol)	E_a (kcal/mol)	Q_{10}	
		20°C → 30°C	60°C → 70°C
50	12	2.0	1.7
85	20	3.1	2.4
100	24	3.9	2.9

In general, the values of E_a range from about 50 to 85 kJ/mol and values above 100 kJ/mol are very uncommon in the pharmaceutical chemistry. Thus, going from room temperature to refrigerator temperature, the value of a first-order rate constant will decrease and the shelf-life increase by a factor of 2 to 4 for every 10°C decrease:

$$k_{T-10} = \frac{k_T}{Q_{10}} \tag{2.107}$$

$$t_{90_{T-10}} = t_{90_T} \cdot Q_{10} \tag{2.108}$$

Likewise, the half-life will increase with decreasing temperature:

$$t_{1/2_{T-10}} = t_{1/2_T} \cdot Q_{10} \tag{2.109}$$

Example 2.10: Shelf-life estimation
A penicillin mixture has a shelf-life of 10 days when stored in the refrigerator (5°C). By mistake, the mixture was stored at room temperature (25°C) for the first 24 hours before it was placed in a refrigerator. How much is the shelf-life reduced?

Answer:

If $Q_{10} = 2$:

$t_{90_{T+20}} = \frac{10 \text{ days}}{2 \cdot 2} = 2.5$ days at 25°C with 1.5 days left at 25°C.

1.5 days at 25°C correspond to $t_{90_{T-20}} = 1.5 \cdot 2 \cdot 2 = 6$ days.

Total $t_{90} = 1 + 6 = 7$ days. Reduced by 3 days.

If $Q_{10} = 3$:

$t_{90_{T+20}} = \frac{10 \text{ days}}{3 \cdot 3} = 1.1$ days at 25°C with 0.1 days left at 25°C.

0.1 days at 25°C correspond to $t_{90_{T-20}} = 0.1 \cdot 3 \cdot 3 = 1$ day.

Total $t_{90} = 1 + 1 = 2$ days. Reduced by 8 days.

If $Q_{10} = 4$:

$t_{90_{T+20}} = \frac{10 \text{ days}}{4 \cdot 4} = 0.6$ days at 25°C with 0 days left at 25°C.

Reduced by 9 days.

Example 2.11: Prolonging shelf-life by storage in refrigerator
An aqueous drug solution was prepared in a hospital pharmacy and the shelf-life is known to be 7 days when the solution is stored at room temperature (25°C). Estimate the shelf-life when the solution is stored at 15°C (cold room) and at 8°C (refrigerator).

Answer:

If $Q_{10} = 2$:

At 15°C $t_{90_{T-10}} = 7 \cdot 2 = 14$ days. At 5°C $t_{90_{T-20}} = 7 \cdot 2 \cdot 2 = 28$ days.

If $Q_{10} = 3$:

At 15°C $t_{90_{T-10}} = 7 \cdot 3 = 21$ day. At 5°C $t_{90_{T-20}} = 7 \cdot 3 \cdot 3 = 63$ days.

If $Q_{10} = 4$:

At 15°C $t_{90_{T-10}} = 7 \cdot 4 = 28$ days. At 5°C $t_{90_{T-20}} = 7 \cdot 4 \cdot 4 = 112$ days.

Thus, the shelf-life will be increased from 7 days to at least 1 month if the solution is stored in a refrigerator.

2.7.2 The Effect of Temperature on Equilibrium Constants

The effect of temperature on an equilibrium constant is given by:

$$A \underset{\longleftarrow}{\overset{K}{\longrightarrow}} B \tag{2.110}$$

$$\Delta G° = -RT\ln K \tag{2.111}$$

$\Delta G°$ is the standard change of free energy of the equilibrium, R is the gas constant, and T is the absolute temperature. Eq. 2.111 can be rearranged to:

$$K = e^{-\frac{\Delta G°}{RT}} \tag{2.112}$$

Furthermore, since the relationship between change in Gibbs free energy (ΔG), change in enthalpy (ΔH), and change in entropy (ΔS) is given by:

$$\Delta G = \Delta H - T\Delta S \tag{2.113}$$

the following equation is obtained by combining Eqs. 2.112 and 2.113:

$$K = e^{-\frac{\Delta H°}{RT}} \times e^{\frac{\Delta S°}{R}} \tag{2.114}$$

or

$$\ln K = -\frac{\Delta H°}{R} \cdot \frac{1}{T} + \frac{\Delta S°}{R} \tag{2.115}$$

A plot of $\ln K$ vs T^{-1} gives a straight line where $\Delta H°$ is obtained from the slope and $\Delta S°$ from the intercept. Eq. 2.115 is a form of the van 't Hoff equation, as is Eq. 2.116:

$$\ln\frac{K_2}{K_1} = \frac{\Delta H°}{R}\left(\frac{T_2 - T_1}{T_1 T_2}\right) \tag{2.116}$$

2.7.3 Transition-State Theory and Eyring Equation

According to the transition-state theory, a quasi-equilibrium exists between the reactants and an activated complex called *transition state* ($[A - B]^{\neq}$), a state at the highest energy along the reaction coordinate (Fig. 2.9) [12].

The equilibrium constant for the transition state is:

$$K^{\neq} = \frac{[A \cdot B]^{\neq}}{[A][B]} \tag{2.117}$$

or

$$[A \cdot B]^{\neq} = K^{\neq}[A][B] \tag{2.118}$$

The rate of a bimolecular reaction shown in Fig. 2.9 will then be:

$$-\frac{d[A]}{dt} = \upsilon K^{\neq}[A][B] = k[A][B] \tag{2.119}$$

where υ is the frequency of the transition state forming the product (P). The rate constant is:

$$k = \upsilon K^{\neq} \tag{2.120}$$

The frequency factor is given by:

$$\upsilon = \frac{RT}{Nh} \tag{2.121}$$

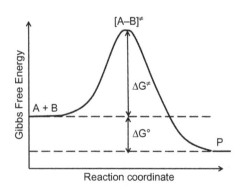

$$A + B \underset{}{\overset{K^{\neq}}{\rightleftharpoons}} [A–B]^{\neq} \longrightarrow P$$

Figure 2.9 Reaction coordinate diagram for a bimolecular reaction where $[A - B]^{\neq}$ represents the transition state.

where R is the gas constant, T is the absolute temperature, N is Avogadro's number, and h is Plank's constant. $K^{\neq}$ is expressed in terms of $\Delta G^{\neq}$ (see Fig. 2.9):

$$\Delta G^{\neq} = \Delta G°(\text{transition state}) - \Delta G°(\text{reactants})$$

$\Delta G^{\neq}$ is closely related to the activation energy (E_a) for the reaction and represents the minimum energy the reactants must acquire for the reaction to take place. As in the previous section (2.7.1), the following equation can be solved for the transition state:

$$\Delta G^{\neq} = -RT \ln K^{\neq} \tag{2.122}$$

$$K^{\neq} = e^{-\frac{\Delta G^{\neq}}{RT}} \tag{2.123}$$

$$K^{\neq} = e^{-\frac{\Delta H^{\neq}}{RT}} \cdot e^{\frac{\Delta S^{\neq}}{R}} \tag{2.124}$$

Combining Eqs. 2.120, 2.121, and 2.124 gives:

$$k = \frac{RT}{Nh} \cdot e^{\frac{\Delta S^{\neq}}{R}} \cdot e^{-\frac{\Delta H^{\neq}}{RT}} \tag{2.125}$$

Eq. 2.125 is related to Eqs. 2.100 and 2.101 where

$$Z = \frac{RT}{Nh} \tag{2.126}$$

and

$$P = e^{\frac{\Delta S^{\neq}}{R}} \tag{2.127}$$

Analogous to the Arrhenius equation (Eq. 2.101), the transition state theory, gives:

$$k = PZe^{-\frac{\Delta H^{\neq}}{RT}} \tag{2.128}$$

The Eyring equation is obtained from Eq. 2.125:

$$\frac{k}{T} = \frac{R}{Nh} \cdot e^{\frac{\Delta S^{\neq}}{R}} \cdot e^{-\frac{\Delta H^{\neq}}{RT}} \tag{2.129}$$

or

$$\ln \frac{k}{T} = \ln\left(\frac{R}{Nh}\right) + \frac{\Delta S^{\neq}}{R} - \frac{\Delta H^{\neq}}{R} \cdot \frac{1}{T} \tag{2.130}$$

A typical Eyring plot is displayed in Fig. 2.10.

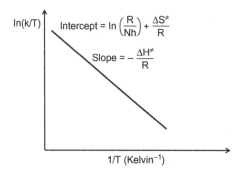

Figure 2.10 Eyring plot used to determine $\Delta H^{\neq}$ from the slope and $\Delta S^{\neq}$ from the intercept.

Example 2.12: Determination of $\Delta H^{\neq}$ and $\Delta S^{\neq}$

Atropine is an ester that is hydrolyzed in aqueous solutions. In Example 2.9 and 2.10, the activation energy was calculated to be 68.08 kJ/mol (16.27 kcal/mol). Calculate $\Delta H^{\neq}$ and $\Delta S^{\neq}$.

Answer:

First, we need to convert the data from the table in Example 2.9 and 2.10 to the Y ($\ln(k/T)$) and X ($1/T$) values of Eq. 2.130:

Temperature (°C)	Temperature (K)	1/T (K⁻¹)	k (min⁻¹)	k/T (K⁻¹ min⁻¹)	ln(k/T)
60	333.15	$3.002 \ 10^{-3}$	$8.45 \ 10^{-6}$	$2.536 \ 10^{-8}$	-17.490
50	323.15	$3.095 \ 10^{-3}$	$3.94 \ 10^{-6}$	$1.220 \ 10^{-8}$	-18.222
40	313.15	$3.193 \ 10^{-3}$	$1.77 \ 10^{-6}$	$5.637 \ 10^{-9}$	-18.994

Then the data is plotted according to Eq. 2.130:

$$\text{ln}(k/T)$$

$$\text{Intercept} = \ln\left(\frac{R}{Nh}\right) + \frac{\Delta S^{\neq}}{R} = 6.1490$$

$$\text{Slope} = -\frac{\Delta H^{\neq}}{R} = -7874.37 \text{ K}$$

$$1/T \text{ (Kelvin}^{-1})$$

$$\text{Intercept} = \ln\left(\frac{R}{Nh}\right) + \frac{\Delta S^{\neq}}{R} \quad \text{or} \quad \frac{\Delta S^{\neq}}{R} = \text{Intercept} - \ln\left(\frac{R}{Nh}\right)$$

$$\frac{\Delta S^{\neq}}{R} = 6.1490 - \ln\left(\frac{8.3143 (\text{J mol}^{-1}\text{K}^{-1})}{6.022 \cdot 10^{23}(\text{mol}^{-1})\, 6.6262 \cdot 10^{34}(\text{J s})\, 60^{-1}(\text{min s}^{-1})}\right)$$

The unit of k/T is $\text{K}^{-1}\,\text{min}^{-1}$ and the units of (R/Nh) must be the identical to those before taking the logarithm. Thus, we needed to convert seconds to minutes in the above equation.

$$\frac{\Delta S^{\neq}}{R} = 6.1490 - 27.8543 = -21.7053$$

$$R = 8.3143 \text{ J mol}^{-1}\,\text{K}^{-1} = 1.9872 \text{ cal}^{-1}\,\text{mol}^{-1}\,\text{K}^{-1}$$

$$\Delta S^{\neq} = -21.7053 \times R = -180.5 \text{ J mol}^{-1}\,\text{K}^{-1} = -43.13 \text{ cal mol}^{-1}\,\text{K}^{-1}$$

$$\text{Slope} = -\frac{\Delta H^{\neq}}{R} = -7874.37 \text{ K}$$

$$-\Delta H^{\neq} = -7874.37 \text{ K} \times R \Rightarrow \Delta H^{\neq} = 65.47 \text{ kJ mol}^{-1} = 15.65 \text{ kcal mol}^{-1}$$

It can be seen that $\Delta H^{\neq} \approx E_a$. Then $\Delta G^{\neq}$ can be calculated according to Eq. 2.113:

$$\Delta G^{\neq} = \Delta H^{\neq} - T\Delta S^{\neq} = 65470 \text{ (J mol}^{-1}) - 298.15 \text{ (K)}$$
$$\times -180.5 \text{ (J mol}^{-1}\text{K}^{-1}) \Rightarrow$$
$$\Delta G^{\neq} = 119286 \text{ J mol}^{-1} = 119.3 \text{ kJ mol}^{-1} \text{ at } 25°C \text{ (298.15 K)}$$

2.8 SPECIFIC ACID/BASE CATALYSIS AND pH-RATE PROFILES

The hydronium ion, most often represented by H^+ or H_3O^+, and the hydroxide ion, OH^-, catalyze drug degradation in aqueous solutions. When H^+ catalyzes a reaction it is called *specific acid catalysis*, when OH^- catalyzes the reaction it is called *specific base catalysis*, and when neither H^+ nor OH^- catalyzes the reaction it is called *solvent catalysis*. The concentrations of H^+ and OH^- vary considerably with pH, and frequently drugs display a pH of maximum stability. For example, ethyl *p*-hydroxybenzoate (ethyl paraben) is an ester that is hydrolyzed in aqueous solution to form *p*-hydroxybenzoic acid and ethanol. Ethyl *p*-hydroxybenzoate is a phenol with a pKa of about 9 at room temperature [13]. Each of the two ionization forms (i.e., EH and E^-) can undergo specific acid catalyzed hydrolysis (rate constant

k_H), solvent catalyzed hydrolysis (rate constant k_0), and specific base catalyzed hydrolysis (rate constant k_{OH}):

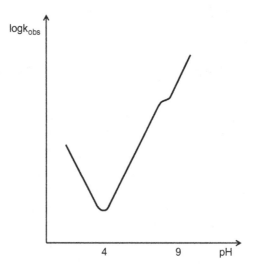

We regard the two ionization forms as separate compounds, with independent rate constants, although in equilibrium with each other. The pH-rate profile was determined in an aqueous solution (Fig. 2.11).

The profile shows that below pH 4, the rate increases as $[H^+]$ increases, and above pH 4, the rate increases as $[OH^-]$ increases. Also, a break in the straight line is observed at $pH \approx pK_a$. Eq. 2.131 contains all six possible reaction rate functions:

$$-\frac{d[E]_T}{dt} = k_H[H^+][EH] + k_0[EH] + [OH^-][EH] + k'_H[H^+][E^-]$$
$$+ k'_0[E^-] + k'_{OH}[OH^-][E^-]$$
(2.131)

Figure 2.11 Sketch of the pH–logk$_{obs}$ profile of ethyl p-hydroxybenzoate in aqueous solution. Notice that since pH is based on the common logarithm (pH ≈ −log[H⁺]) logk$_{obs}$ is plotted on the Y-axis.

where $[E]_T$ is the total concentration of ethyl p-hydroxybenzoate:

$$[E]_T = [EH] + [E^-] \tag{2.132}$$

From the profile displayed in Fig. 2.11, we can clearly observe k_H at pH below 4, k_{OH} at pH between about 4 and 9, and k'_{OH} at pH above 9. It is also quite possible that k_0 is present at pH of about 4. However, k'_H and k'_0 cannot be observed. Thus, the corresponding functions in Eq. 2.131 can be deleted:

$$-\frac{d[E]_T}{dt} = k_H[H^+][EH] + k_0[EH] + k_{OH}[OH^-][EH] + k'_{OH}[OH^-][E^-] \tag{2.133}$$

At pH $<$ 4 Eq. 2.133 becomes:

$$-\frac{d[E]_T}{dt} \approx k_H[H^+][EH] \tag{2.134}$$

and since pH $\approx -\log[H^+]$, the slope of the profile should theoretically be close to -1. At pH between about 4 and 9, Eq. 2.133 approaches

$$-\frac{d[E]_T}{dt} \approx k_{OH}[OH^-][EH] \tag{2.135}$$

and since pH $\approx -\log(K_w/[OH^-])$, the slope of the profile should theoretically be close to $+1$. At pH $>$ 9, Eq. 2.133 approaches:

$$-\frac{d[E]_T}{dt} \approx k'_{OH}[OH^-][E^-] \tag{2.136}$$

and, again, the slope should be close to $+1$. If k_o has a relatively large value, the minimum of the pH $-$ logk_{obs} profile will display a plateau, but it will be sharp if k_o is relatively small:

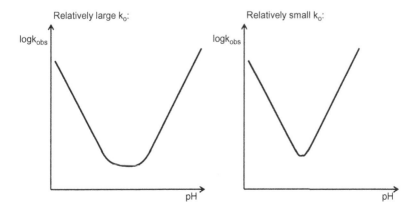

It can also be seen that:

$$f_{EH} = \frac{[EH]}{[EH] + [E^-]} = \frac{[H^+]}{[H^+] + K_a} \qquad (2.137)$$

and

$$f_{E^-} = \frac{[E^-]}{[EH] + [E^-]} = \frac{K_a}{[H^+ + K_a]} \qquad (2.138)$$

and furthermore, that $[EH] = f_{EH} \cdot [E]_T$ and $[E^-] = f_{E^-} \cdot [E]_T$. Thus, Eq. 2.131 can be written as:

$$-\frac{d[E]_T}{dt} = \left(k_H [H^+] f_{EH} + k_0 f_{EH} + k_{OH}[OH^-] f_{EH} + k'_{OH}[OH^-] f_{E^-} \right)[E]_T$$

$$(2.139)$$

where k_{obs} in Fig. 2.11 is

$$k_{obs} = \left(k_H[H^+] f_{EH} + k_0 f_{EH} + k_{OH}[OH^-] f_{EH} + k'_{OH}[OH^-] f_{E^-} \right) \quad (2.140)$$

and

$$-\frac{d[E]_T}{dt} = k_{obs}[E]_T \qquad (2.141)$$

Example 2.13: Specific acid and specific base catalysis
The figure below shows the pH-rate profile for ester hydrolysis at 60°C. Estimate the values of k_H, k_0, and k_{OH}. k_{obs} is in min^{-1} and pK_w is 13.02 at 60°C.

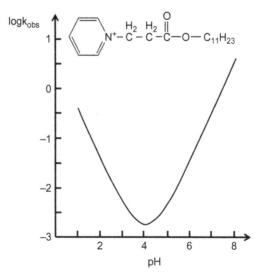

Answer:

At pH = 1.0 [H$^+$] = 0.10 and log$k_{obs} \approx -0.4$ or $k_{obs} \approx 0.4$ min^{-1}:

$$k_{obs} = k_H [H^+] \text{ or } k_H = \frac{k_{obs}}{[H^+]} \approx \frac{0.4}{0.10} = 4.0 \text{ M}^{-1} \text{ min}^{-1}$$

At pH = 8.0 log$k_{obs} \approx 0.5$ or $k_{obs} \approx 3.2$ min^{-1} and [OH$^-$] = 10$^{-(pK_w - pH)}$ = 10$^{-5.02}$

$$k_{obs} = k_{OH}[OH^-] \text{ and, thus, } k_{OH} = \frac{k_{obs}}{[OH^-]} \approx \frac{3.2}{10^{-5.02}} = 3.4 \times 10^5 \text{ M}^{-1}\text{min}^{-1}.$$

From $k_{obs} = k_H[H^+] + k_0 + k_{OH}[OH^-]$ and log$k_{obs} \approx -2.8$ ($k_{obs} \approx 1.6 \times 10^{-3}$ min^{-1}) at pH = 4.0, it can be calculated that $k_0 \approx 8.8 \times 10^{-4}$ min^{-1}.

2.9 GENERAL ACID/BASE CATALYSIS OR BUFFER CATALYSIS

In aqueous solutions, general acid/base catalysis involves acids and bases other than H$^+$ and OH$^-$ (i.e., compounds other than water that are able to donate or accept protons). In pharmaceutical formulations, these proton donors and acceptors are frequently buffer salts and the process is called buffer catalysis. For a simple ester hydrolysis catalyzed by a buffer (B), the rate equation could be:

$$-\frac{d[E]_T}{dt} = k_H [H^+][E] + k_0[E] + k_{OH}[OH^-][E] + k_B[B]_T[E] \quad (2.142)$$

where [B]$_T$ is the total buffer concentration:

$$[B]_T = [BH] + [B^-] \quad (2.143)$$

If k'_{obs} is the observed rate constant when no buffer salts are present, then Eq. 2.142 can be simplified to:

$$-\frac{d[E]_T}{dt} = k'_{obs}[E] + k_B[B]_T[E] \quad (2.144)$$

where

$$k_{obs} = k'_{obs} + k_B[B]_T \quad (2.145)$$

To determine the buffer, catalysis k_{obs} is plotted against $[B]_T$ at a constant pH (i.e., where the total buffer concentration varies, but the molar ratios of the buffer salts are constant):

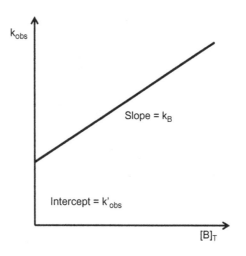

Figure 2.12 Plot according to Eq. 2.145 to determine buffer catalysis.

To determine if the buffer salts are causing general acid or general base catalysis, the buffer catalysis is determined at two slightly different pH values and k_{BH} and k_B are calculated by applying the following equations as shown in Example 2.14:

$$k_{obs} = k'_{obs} + k_{BH}[BH] + k_B[B^-] = k'_{obs} + (k_{BH}f_{BH} + k_B f_B)[B]_T \quad (2.146)$$

where

$$f_{BH} = \frac{[BH]}{[BH] + [B^-]} = \frac{[H^+]}{[H^+] + K_a} \quad (2.147)$$

and

$$f_B = \frac{[B^-]}{[BH] + [B^-]} = \frac{K_a}{[H^+] + K_a} \quad (2.148)$$

Like other reactions, in catalysis, the buffer salts lower the activation energy by providing an alternative reaction route to the products (Fig. 2.13).

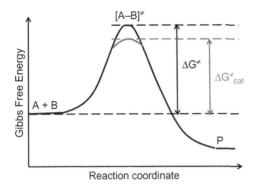

Figure 2.13 Reaction coordinate diagram showing the effect of catalysis on a bimolecular reaction where [A – B]$^{\neq}$ represents the transition state and $\Delta G^{\neq}$ and $\Delta G^{\neq}_{cat}$ the activation energies for the uncatalyzed and the catalyzed reactions, respectively.

Since the transition state is of lower energy in the catalyzed reaction, more reactant molecules have sufficient energy to react and, consequently, the reaction proceeds faster.

Example 2.14: Buffer catalysis

Guo et al. [14] investigated phosphate buffer catalyzed degradation of lithospermic acid B at pH 7.05 and 6.50, I = 0.5, and 90°C, and obtained the following results:

pH	[Phosphate]$_T$	k_{obs} (h^{-1})
7.05	0.192	1.114
	0.096	0.958
	0.048	0.880
6.50	0.192	0.768
	0.096	0.660
	0.048	0.607

Calculate the buffer catalysis (i.e., the general acid catalysis ($k_{H_2PO_4^-}$) and general base catalysis ($k_{HPO_4^{2-}}$)) for the degradation of lithospermic acid B under these conditions. pK_{a2} for phosphoric acid is 7.08 at 90°C.

Answer:

Eq. 2.146: $k_{obs} = k'_{obs} + (k_{BH}f_{BH} + k_B f_B)[B]_T$, where $[B]_T = [Phosphate]_T$

Eq. 2.146 is an equation of a straight line where $(k_{BH}f_{BH} + k_B f_B)$ is the slope and k'_{obs} is the intercept:

$$k_{obs} = k'_{obs} + \left(k_{H_2PO_4^-} \times f_{H_2PO_4^-} + k_{HPO_4^{2-}} \times f_{HPO_4^{2-}} \right) \times [Phosphate]_T$$

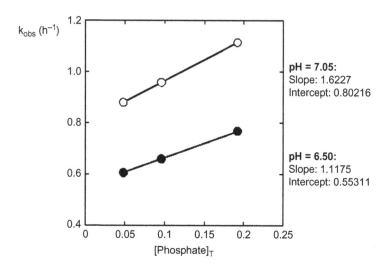

If we know the pH (i.e., $[H^+]$) and the pK_a, we can apply Eq. 2.147 to determine the fraction of the acidic form of the buffer ($H_2PO_4^-$) and Eq. 2.148 to determine the basic form of the buffer (HPO_4^{2-}).

pH 7.05:

$$k_{obs} = 0.80216 + 1.6227 \times [P]_T$$

$$f_{H_2PO_4^-} = \frac{[H^+]}{[H^+] + K_{a2}} = \frac{10^{-7.05}}{10^{-7.05} + 10^{-7.08}} = 0.5173$$

$$f_{HPO_4^{2-}} = \frac{[H^+]}{[H^+] + K_{a2}} = \frac{10^{-7.08}}{10^{-7.05} + 10^{-7.08}} = 0.4827$$

pH 6.50:

$$k_{obs} = 0.55311 + 1.1175 \times [P]_T$$

$$f_{H_2PO_4^-} = \frac{[H^+]}{[H^+] + K_{a2}} = \frac{10^{-6.50}}{10^{-6.50} + 10^{-7.08}} = 0.7917$$

$$f_{HPO_4^{2-}} = \frac{[H^+]}{[H^+] + K_{a2}} = \frac{10^{-7.08}}{10^{-6.50} + 10^{-7.08}} = 0.2083$$

pH 7.05: $1.6227 \ M^{-1} \ h^{-1} = k_{H_2PO_4} \ 0.5173 + k_{HPO_4} \ 0.4827$

pH 6.50: $1.1175 \ M^{-1} \ h^{-1} = k_{H_2PO_4} \ 0.7917 + k_{HPO_4} \ 0.2083$

Solved together, the two equations give $k_{HPO_4} = 2.578 \ M^{-1} \ h^{-1}$ and $k_{H_2PO_4} = 0.734 \ M^{-1} \ h^{-1}$

Thus, the general base catalysis is dominating, although some general acid catalysis is also observed.

2.10 EFFECTS OF IONIC STRENGTH (SALT EFFECTS)

If the drug is ionized, the reaction rate is influenced by electrostatic interactions between the drug and other reacting ions, as well as by the ionic strength of the aqueous reaction medium. The ions attract or repel each other as well as affect the water structure and hydration of dissolved molecules and transition states. These effects are called *ionic strength effects* or *salt effects* and are of two types, primary and secondary salt effects.

Ionic strength (I) of an aqueous solution is a measure of the ionic concentration:

$$I = \frac{1}{2} \sum (mz^2) = \frac{1}{2}\left(m_A z_A^2 + m_B z_B^2 + m_C z_C^2 + \ldots\right) \tag{2.149}$$

where m is the molality (moles per kg solvent), but using molarity (moles per liter solution) for aqueous solutions at room temperature does not cause significant error. The density of liquid water is close to unity at and below room temperature (e.g., 1.000; 0.997; and 0.992 g/ml at 10, 25, and 40°C, respectively, and 1 atm). z is the electric charge. For example, if 9.0 g NaCl (MW 58.44 g/mol) is dissolved in one liter of pure water (i.e., isotonic saline solution) the concentration of the two ions will be:

$$[Na^+] = [Cl^-] = 9.0/55.44 = 0.162 \, mol/liter$$

and the ionic strength of the solution will be:

$$I = \tfrac{1}{2}(0.162 \cdot (+1)^2 + 0.162 \cdot (-1)^2) = 0.16 \, mol/kg$$

Almost all pharmaceutical solutions are rather concentrated solutions of one or more active ingredient and pharmaceutical excipients. These are nonideal solutions and, thus, deviate from ideal behavior. To correct for their nonideality, *activity* (a) is used to measure "effective concentration" of different solution species. The *chemical potential* of a drug in a nonideal solution, depends on the activity (a) in the same way that it depends on the drug concentration in ideal solutions. The activity is proportional to the concentration:

$$a = \gamma \cdot [A] \tag{2.150}$$

where the proportional constant is the *activity constant* (γ) and [A] is the molal concentration of A, but for all practical purposes the molality (moles per kg solvent) can be replaced by the molarity (moles per liter solution). The activity coefficient of a given ion (γ_i) in a dilute aqueous solution is given by the Debye-Hückel equation ($I < 0.01 \, mol/kg$ and $25°C$):

$$\log\gamma_i = -0.51z_i^2\sqrt{I} \tag{2.151}$$

2.10.1 Primary Salt Effect

Primary salt effects are observed when the added salts do not have a direct catalytic effect on the reaction and do not have any ions in common with the drug or other reactants. The observed affect on the reaction rate is then due to changes in the activity coefficient (γ) as a result of changes in the ionic strength of the reaction medium (see Fig. 2.9):

$$A + B \underset{\longleftarrow}{\overset{K^{\neq}}{\longrightarrow}} [A-B]^{\neq} \to P$$

The equilibrium constant for the transition state was given by Eq. 2.117 in terms of the concentration of the reacting species.

However, in its more correct form, concentration is replaced by the activity:

$$K^{\neq} = \frac{a^{\neq}_{AB}}{a_A a_B} = \frac{[A \cdot B]^{\neq}}{[A][B]} \cdot \frac{\gamma^{\neq}_{AB}}{\gamma_A \gamma_B} \qquad (2.152)$$

If k_0 is the rate constant in an ideal solution (i.e., a very dilute solution), where $I = 0$, and consequently $\gamma = 1$ (from Eq. 2.151), then from Eqs. 2.119 and 2.152 we get:

$$k = k_0 \frac{\gamma_A \gamma_B}{\gamma^{\neq}_{AB}} \qquad (2.153)$$

Taking the common logarithm of Eq. 2.153, gives:

$$\log k = \log k_0 + \log \gamma_A + \log \gamma_B - \log \gamma^{\neq}_{AB} \qquad (2.154)$$

where

$$\log \gamma^{\neq}_{AB} = -0.51(z_A + z_B)^2 \sqrt{I} \qquad (2.155)$$

$(z_A + z_B)$ is the charge of the transition state (the activated complex). If we combine Eqs. 2.151, 2.154, and 2.155 we get:

$$\log k = \log k_0 - 0.51z_A^2 \sqrt{I} - 0.51z_B^2 \sqrt{I} + 0.51z_A^2 \sqrt{I} + 1.02z_A z_B \sqrt{I}$$
$$+ 0.51z_B^2 \sqrt{I} \qquad (2.156)$$

or

$$\log k = \log k_0 + 1.02z_A z_B \sqrt{I} \qquad (2.157)$$

Eq. 2.157 is reasonably accurate in dilute aqueous solutions and gives some idea of the ionic strength effects in more concentrated solutions. This is due to the fact that Eq. 2.151 is a simplification of more complex relationships that are observed in more concentrated aqueous solutions. Eq. 2.158 (the Brønsted-Bjerrum equation) is a slightly more accurate equation, but still only applicable in relatively dilute solutions:

$$\log k = \log k_0 + 1.02z_A z_B \frac{\sqrt{I}}{1 + \sqrt{I}} \qquad (2.158)$$

$$A + B \xrightarrow{\ k\ } P \qquad (2.159)$$

Theoretically, when molecules A and B react (Eq. 2.159), the rate constant (k) will increase with increasing ionic strength (I) if A and B have the same charge, but k will decrease with an increasing I if A and B have different charges. If A or B, or both A and B, are uncharged, k should not be affected by changes in I. However, changes in I will, in general, result in some changes in k, even when the reactants (A and/or B) are uncharged.

Since the pH-scale and the pK_a values are based on the common logarithm, it is customary to use it (and not the natural logarithm) in calculations that relate to pH and pK_a values.

2.10.2 Secondary Salt Effect

Changes in I can also change the ionization constants (K_a) of weak acids and bases, and thereby the concentrations of H^+ and OH^-. Since reaction rates depend upon H^+ and OH^- concentrations (see section 2.8), the rates will be affected by I. This phenomenon is known as the *secondary salt effect*. At relatively low ionic strength ($I < 0.3$), the following can be used to determine the apparent dissociation constant (pK'_a) at a given I:

$$pK'_a = pK_a + \frac{0.51(2z - 1)\sqrt{I}}{1 + \sqrt{I}} \qquad (2.160)$$

where pK_a is the dissociation constant in an ideal (i.e., very dilute) solution (i.e., thermodynamic dissociation constant) and z is the charge of the acid.

Example 2.15: Dissociation constant of aspirin
Calculate the apparent dissociation constant of aspirin (acetylsalicylic acid) in an isotonic saline solution (i.e., aqueous 0.9% w/v NaCl solution) at 25°C. pK_a of aspirin is 3.485 at 25°C.

Answer:

The molecular weight of NaCl is 58.44 g/mol and, thus, the ionic strength of the solution is calculated as follows:

$$[Na^+] = [Cl^-] = 9.0/55.44 = 0.162 \text{ mol/liter}$$

$$I = \frac{1}{2}(0.162 \cdot (+1)^2 + 0.162 \cdot (-1)^2) = 0.16 \text{ mol/kg}$$

Then we use Eq. 2.160 to calculate the apparent dissociation constant (pK'_a) at $I = 0.16 \, mol/kg$, noting that the acid form of aspirin is uncharged ($z = 0$):

$$pK'_a = pK_a + \frac{0.51(2z-1)\sqrt{I}}{1+\sqrt{I}} = 3.485 + \frac{0.51(2 \times 0 - 1)\sqrt{0.16}}{1+\sqrt{0.16}}$$

$$= 3.485 - \frac{0.51 \times \sqrt{0.16}}{1+\sqrt{0.16}} = 3.485 - 0.146 = 3.34$$

Thus, the apparent K_a increases from 3.27×10^{-4} to 4.57×10^{-4} (i.e., aspirin becomes a slightly stronger acid in saline).

2.11 SOLVENT EFFECTS

Frequently, pharmaceutical formulations consist of aqueous solutions containing not only water, but also organic solvents such as ethanol and glycerol. The addition of organic solvents to aqueous drug solutions will change the *dielectric constant* (ε) of the solution media and, thus, the ability of the media to stabilize (or destabilize) the transition state (see section 2.7.2):

$$A + B \underset{\longleftarrow}{\overset{K^{\neq}}{\longrightarrow}} [A-B]^{\neq} \rightarrow P$$

Solvents composed of polar molecules like water will generally be in random orientations but will take on an ordered orientation when an electric field is applied to the solvent. In polar molecules, positive and negative charges are distributed unevenly. Such molecules are said to be polar and to possess dipole moments. Polar solvent molecules will orientate their positive charges toward negative charges of a solute or a transition state, and their negative charges toward positive charges of a solute or a transition state. Stabilization of a transition state will increase the value of $K^{\neq}$ and, consequently, lead to an increased reaction rate (Eq. 2.120). The dielectric constant is a measure of solvent polarity. It measures the reduction of the field strength of the electric field surrounding a charged particle immersed in a solvent compared to the field strength surrounding the same particle in a vacuum. In general, solvents with $\varepsilon < 15$ are considered nonpolar. At 25°C, the ε of water is 78.5, that of glycerol 42.5, ethanol 24.3, acetone 20.7, and diethyl ether 4.2. If both A and B are ions, with charges z_A and z_B, the following equation can be used to determine the effect of changes in the medium dielectric constant on the reaction rate:

$$\ln k = \ln k_{\varepsilon = \infty} - \frac{K z_A z_B}{\varepsilon} \qquad (2.161)$$

where K is a constant for a given reaction at some given temperature. Theoretically, when molecules A and B react (Eq. 2.161), the rate constant (k) will increase with increasing dielectric constant (ε) if A and B have the same charge, but k will decrease with increasing ε if A and B have different charges (i.e., are unlike-sign ions). If A or B, or both A and B, are uncharged, k should not be affected by changes in ε. However, changes in ε will frequently result in some changes in k, even when the reactants (A and B) are uncharged.

Example 2.16: Degradation of aspartame
The figure below shows the pH-rate profile for the degradation of aspartame at 60°C in water and aqueous ethanol solutions [15]. Describe the effect of the medium dielectric constant on the degradation. How will the addition of ethanol to a soft drink (pH 3.3) affect the stability of aspartame?

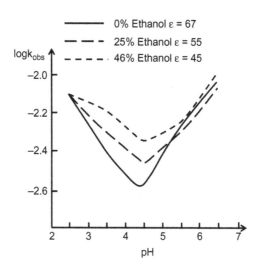

Answer:

Aspartame has two ionizable groups:

The pK_a values for aspartame in pure water at room temperature are approximately 3.1 and 7.9. The sweetener exists predominantly as a cation at a pH below 3, as a zwitterion at a pH between 3 and 8, and as an anion at a pH above 8. The figure shows that changes in ε have a significant effect on the specific acid catalyzed degradation of the zwitterionic form, but much less of an effect on its specific base catalyzed degradation or on the specific acid catalyzed degradation of the cationic form. At a pH between 3 and 4.5, the rate decreases with an increasing ε. According to Eq. 2.161, k_{obs} will decrease with an increasing ε if the reactants (i.e., A and B) have different charges (i.e., negative and positive charges) indicating that the specific acid catalyzed degradation might possibly involve intramolecular catalysis of the carboxylate ion on the protonated ester bond or on the formation of a cyclic intermediate [16]. Specific base catalysis (that could, for example, involve an OH^- attack on the ester bond) is much less affected by changes in ε (since A and B both carry a negative charge). Apparently, the ammonium ion has much less of an effect on the reaction rate than the carboxylate ion does.

The addition of ethanol to a diet soft drink containing aspartame will destabilize the sweetener.

2.12 DISPERSE COLLOIDAL SYSTEMS (MICELLE EFFECT)

Drug incorporation into micelles, liposomes, and other liquid colloidal systems can sometimes decrease drug degradation rate. An oil-in-water emulsion is an example of a colloidal system, a mixture of two liquids

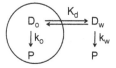

Figure 2.14 Drug degradation within an oil-in-water emulsion.

in which the oil is the lipophilic dispersed phase and water is the aqueous homogeneous phase. In oil-in-water emulsions, drug molecules are distributed between the oil and water (Fig. 2.14).

K_d is the distribution coefficient of the drug between oil and water:

$$K_d = \frac{D_o}{D_w} \qquad (2.162)$$

where D_o is the total amount of dissolved drug located within the oil phase and D_w is the total amount of dissolved drug that is located in the aqueous phase. The observed first-order rate constant for the drug degradation within the oil phase to form product (P) is k_o, and the observed first-order rate constant for drug in the aqueous phase is k_w. The observed first-order rate constant (k_{obs}) for drug degradation within such a system is the weighted average of k_o and k_w:

$$k_{obs} = f_o k_o + f_w k_w \qquad (2.163)$$

$$f_o = \frac{D_o}{D_o + D_w} = \frac{K_d}{1 + K_d} \qquad (2.164)$$

and

$$f_w = \frac{1}{1 + K_d} \qquad (2.165)$$

Example 2.17: Etoposide degradation in emulsion
Etoposide is a hydrophilic anticancer drug with a poor aqueous solubility (0.15 mg/ml). An aqueous etoposide oil-in-water emulsion (20% w/v oil in water) was prepared and the pH-rate profile was determined at a zero buffer concentration and 80°C (k_{obs} is in h^{-1}) [17]:

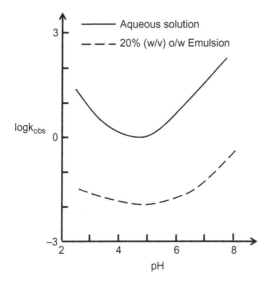

In an emulsion containing 0.1% (w/v) etoposide, about 99% of the drug was estimated to be located in the oil phase, mainly at the oil/water interface, and about 1% in the aqueous solution. At pH 5 and 80°C, the k_{obs} was determined to be 1.08 h^{-1} in the aqueous buffer solution and 1.28×10^{-2} h^{-1} in the emulsion. Estimate k_o and k_w. Discuss the observed changes in the pH-rate profile upon introduction of oil into the medium.

Answer:

The value of k_w is equal to k_{obs} at pH 5 ($k_{obs} = 1.08$ h^{-1}). $f_o \approx 0.99$ and $f_w \approx 0.01$. Inserting these values into Eq. 2.163 gives

$$1.28 \times 10^{-2} h^{-1} = 0.99 \times k_o + 0.01 \times 1.08\ h^{-1}$$

or $k_o \approx 2.0 \times 10^{-3}$ h^{-1} at 80°C. It can also be seen that

$$K_d = \frac{D_o}{D_w} \approx 100$$

The pH-rate profile in an aqueous buffer solution displays typical specific acid/base catalysis (i.e., slopes of -1 and $+1$). However, in the emulsion, the pH-rate profile does not appear to display typical specific acid catalysis (i.e., the slope at pH < 5 is > -1). Formulating the drug as an o/w parenteral emulsion, results in a 100- to 1000-fold increase in the shelf-life (at 80°C) when compared with its shelf-life in an aqueous solution.

2.13 EFFECT OF COMPLEXATION

Complex formation between drug and excipients (e.g., cyclodextrins, water-soluble polymers, or polyalcohols) or impurities (e.g., metal ions) can lead to the stabilization or destabilization of drugs. The complex formation is a reversible process in which substrate molecules (i.e., drug molecules) associate with ligand molecules (e.g., cyclodextrin (CD) molecules) to form a complex (D/CD). In general, the substrate and ligand are kept together by relatively weak noncovalent forces such as hydrogen bonding, van der Waals forces, electrostatic interactions, and hydrophobic interactions. Here we use cyclodextrin as an example of a ligand. In aqueous cyclodextrin solutions, free drug molecules are in dynamic equilibrium with drug molecules bound within the cyclodextrin complex:

$$
\begin{array}{c}
\ \ \ \ \ \ \ \ \ \ k_c \\
D + CD \rightleftharpoons D/CD \\
\downarrow k_f \ \ \ \ \ \ \ \downarrow k_c
\end{array}
$$

K_c is the stability constant of the complex and k_f and k_c are the first-order rate constants for the free unbound drug and bound drug in the complex, respectively. The observed first-order rate constant (k_{obs}) for the drug degradation is the weighted average of k_f and k_w:

$$k_{obs} = f_f k_f + f_c k_c \tag{2.166}$$

If one drug molecule forms a complex with one cyclodextrin molecule, then the total drug concentration ($[D]_T$) is the sum of the concentration of the free drug ($[D]$) and the concentration of the complex drug ($[D/CD]$), the following equations are obtained:

$$[D]_T = [D] + [D/CD] \tag{2.167}$$

$$[CD]_T = [CD] + [D/CD] \tag{2.168}$$

$$K_{1:1} = \frac{[D/CD]}{[D] \cdot [CD]} \tag{2.169}$$

$$f_f = \frac{[D]}{[D] + [D/CD]} = \frac{1}{1 + K_{1:1} \cdot [CD]} \tag{2.170}$$

$$f_c = 1 - f_f = \frac{K_{1:1} \cdot [CD]}{1 + K_{1:1} \cdot [CD]} \tag{2.171}$$

$$k_{obs} = \frac{k_f + k_c \cdot K_{1:1} \cdot [CD]}{1 + K_{1:1} \cdot [CD]} \tag{2.172}$$

$$-\frac{d[D]_T}{dt} = k_{obs} \cdot [D]_T = \left(\frac{k_f + k_c \cdot K_{1:1} \cdot [CD]}{1 + K_{1:1} \cdot [CD]}\right) \cdot [D]_T \tag{2.173}$$

where $K_{1:1}$ is the stability constant of the 1:1 D/CD complex. If the total cyclodextrin concentration is much greater than the total drug concentration, then it can be assumed that $[CD] \approx [CD]_T$:

$$k_{obs} = \left(\frac{k_f + k_c \cdot K_{1:1} \cdot [CD]_T}{1 + K_{1:1} \cdot [CD]_T}\right) \tag{2.174}$$

Equation 2.174 can then be rearranged into different formats, including that of the Lineweaver-Burk plot where $(k_f - k_{obs})^{-1}$ v $([CD]_T)^{-1}$ will give a straight line from which k_c can be obtained from the intercept and $K_{1:1}$ from the slope:

$$\frac{1}{k_f - k_{obs}} = \frac{1}{K_{1:1} \cdot (k_f - k_c)} \cdot \frac{1}{[CD]_T} + \frac{1}{k_f - k_c} \tag{2.175}$$

Alternatively, k_c and $K_{1:1}$ can be obtained by a simple nonlinear fitting of k_{obs} according to Eq. 2.174. In general, ligands such as cyclodextrins enhance drug stability ($k_f > k_c$), but ligands such as metal ions catalyze drug degradation ($k_f < k_c$).

Example 2.18: Effect of cyclodextrin complexation
The degradation of estramustine was determined in aqueous solutions at pH 7.4 and 80°C [18]. The table below shows the effect of 2-hydroxypropyl-β-cyclodextrin (HPβCD) on the observed degradation rate constant. Calculate k_c and $K_{1:1}$.

[HPβCD] (M)	k_{obs} (min^{-1})
0.000	1.49×10^{-2}
0.007	1.33×10^{-2}
0.014	1.25×10^{-2}
0.022	1.20×10^{-2}
0.036	1.13×10^{-2}
0.073	1.04×10^{-2}

Answer:

We apply Eq. 2.175: $\dfrac{1}{k_f - k_{obs}} = \dfrac{1}{K_{1:1} \cdot (k_f - k_c)} \cdot \dfrac{1}{[CD]_T} + \dfrac{1}{k_f - k_c}$

[HPβCD] (M)	[HPβCD]$_T^{-1}$ (M^{-1})	k_{obs} (min^{-1})	$(k_f\text{-}k_{obs})^{-1}$ (min)
0.000	–	1.49×10^{-2}	–
0.007	142.9	1.33×10^{-2}	625
0.014	71.4	1.25×10^{-2}	417
0.022	45.5	1.20×10^{-2}	345
0.036	27.8	1.13×10^{-2}	278
0.073	13.7	1.04×10^{-2}	222

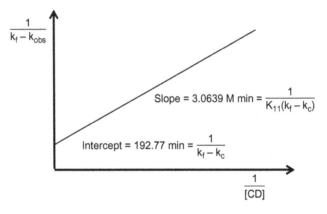

$K_{1:1}$ = Intercept ÷ Slope = 192.77 min ÷ 3.0639 M min = 62.9 M^{-1} at pH 7.4 and 80°C

$k_f = 1.49 \times 10^{-2}$ min^{-1}

192.77 min = $(1.49 \times 10^{-2} - k_c)^{-1} \Rightarrow k_c = 9.71 \times 10^{-3}$ min^{-1} at pH 7.4 and 80°C

Question 2.1: When injected into HPLC, why are the retention times of the drug and the drug/cyclodextrin complex identical? Why do the drug and the complex not give two separate peaks?

2.14 EFFECT OF LIGHT (PHOTODEGRADATION) AND OXYGEN

Light can enhance drug degradation. *Photodegradation* is initiated by absorption of photons of infrared, visible, and ultraviolet light and

other forms of electromagnetic radiation. A drug molecule forms at
the so-called excited state (D*) upon absorption of a photon of light:

$$D \xrightarrow{\text{h}\nu} [D]^* \to P$$

where h is Planck's constant, ν is the frequency of light, the product
(hν) is the energy of a photon, and P is the degradation product.
Sometimes an excipient (or another component of the system) may
absorb photons and then transfer the energy to the active ingredient to
form D*. The frequency depends on the light wavelength (λ):

$$\nu = \frac{c}{\lambda} \tag{2.176}$$

where c is the speed of light. Blue light (a short wavelength) consists of
high energy photons, and red light (a long wavelength) consists of low
energy photons. Consequently, drugs and drug products are, in general,
more sensitive toward blue and ultraviolet light than to red light.
However, drugs possess different absorption spectra and, thus, the rate of
photodegradation depends on the overlap of the absorption spectrum of a
given drug with the spectral distribution of light striking the drug product.

Oxygen availability can affect drug oxidation and frequently drug
degradation rate is proportional to the oxygen concentration:

$$-\frac{d[D]}{dt} = k[D][O_2] = k_{obs}[D] \tag{2.177}$$

Under such conditions, protecting the drug product against oxygen
will decrease the drug degradation rate. Oxygen can exist in various
states. The ground state of oxygen is its triplet state ($^3O_2$), but its
excited state is singlet oxygen ($^1O_2$), which is more reactive than the
triplet form:

Triplet   Singlet

Singlet oxygen is highly oxidizing (photooxidation), capable of
oxidizing unsaturated drug moieties. Other oxygen species also exist
(e.g., peroxides), that are capable of reducing or oxidizing drugs and
excipients. Conditions that promote formation of such species (e.g.,
light and metal ions) can enhance oxidative degradation. Light and
metal ions catalyze autoxidation of unsaturated fatty acids.

REFERENCES

[1] J.L. Patel, A.P. Lemberger, The Kinetics of the hydrolysis of homatropine methylbromide and atropine methylbromide, J. Pharm. Sci. 48 (1959) 106–109.

[2] H. Zia, N. Shalchian, F. Borhanian, Kinetics of amoxycillin degradation in aqueous solutions, Can. J. Pharm. Sci. 12 (1977) 80–83.

[3] J. Walker, Method for determining velocities of saponification, Proc. Roy. Soc. London, Ser. A 78 (1906) 157–160.

[4] K.D. Schlecht, C.W. Frank, Tetracycline epimerization kinetics utilizing NMR spectrometry, J. Pharm. Sci. 62 (1973) 258–261.

[5] M.A. Nunes, E. Brochmann-Hanssen, Hydrolysis and epimerization kinetics of pilocarpine in aqueous solution, J. Pharm. Sci. 63 (1974) 716–721.

[6] H. Bundgaard, S.H. Hansen, Hydrolysis and epimerization kinetics of pilocarpine in basic aqueous solution as determined by HPLC, Int. J. Pharm. 10 (1982) 281–289.

[7] T. Loftsson, N. Bodor, Improved delivery through biological membranes IX: kinetics and mechanism of hydrolysis of methylsulfinylmethyl 2-acetoxybenzoate and related aspirin prodrugs, J. Pharm. Sci. 70 (1981) 750–755.

[8] T. Loftsson, H. Gudmundmiddottir, J.F. Sigurjonmiddottir, H.H. Sigurdsson, S.D. Sigfusson, M. Masson, E. Stefansson, Cyclodextrin solubilization of benzodiazepines: formulation of midazolam nasal spray, Int. J. Pharm. 212 (2001) 29–40.

[9] P. Zvirblis, I. Socholitsky, A.A. Kondritzer, Kinetics of the hydrolysis of atropine, J. Pharm. Sci. 45 (1956) 450–454.

[10] A.A. Kondritzer, P. Zvirblis, Stability of atropine in aqueous solution, J. Pharm. Sci. 46 (1957) 531–535.

[11] K.A. Connors, G.L. Amidon, V.J. Stella, Chemical Stability of Pharmaceuticals: A handbook for pharmacists, John Wiley & Sons, New York, 1986.

[12] K.J. Laidler, M.C. King, The development of transition state theory, J. Phys. Chem. 87 (1983) 2657–2664.

[13] V.B. Sunderland, D.W. Watts, Kinetics of the degradation of methyl, ethyl and n-propyl 4-hydroxybenzoate esters in aqueous solution, Int. J. Pharm. 19 (1984) 1–15.

[14] Y.-X. Guo, Z.-L. Xiu, D.-J. Zhang, H. Wang, L.-X. Wang, H.-B. Xiao, Kinetics and mechanism of degradation of lithospermic acid B in aqueous solution, J. Pharm. Biom. Anal. 43 (2007) 1249–1255.

[15] S. Sanyude, R.A. Locock, L.A. Pagliaro, Stability of aspartame in water:organic solvent mixtures with different dielectric constants, J. Pharm. Sci. 80 (1991) 674–676.

[16] S. Sabah, G.K.E. Scriba, Determination of aspartame and its degradation and epimerization products by capillary electrophoresis, J. Pharm. Biomed. Anal. 16 (1998) 1089–1096.

[17] L. Tian, H. He, X. Tang, Stability and degradation kinetics of etoposide-loaded parenteral lipid emulsion, J. Pharm. Sci. 96 (2007) 1719–1728.

[18] T. Loftsson, B.J. Olafmiddottir, J. Baldvinmiddottir, Estramustine: hydrolysis, solubilization, and stabilization in aqueous solutions, Int. J. Pharm. 79 (1992) 107–112.

CHAPTER 3

Degradation Pathways

3.1 HYDROLYSIS

Hydrolysis indicates cleavage of chemical bonds by the addition of water. Hydrolysis is one of the most common drug degradation reactions, even in solid dosage forms in the presence of moisture, and the most common substrates are those that contain the acyl group:

$R-\overset{\overset{\displaystyle O}{\|}}{C}-X$	X		
Ester	-OR'	Lactone	
Thioester	-SR'		
Amide	-NHR'		
Acid chloride	-Cl	Lactam	
Acid anhydride	-OCOR'		
Imide	-NHCOR'		

Other substrates susceptible to hydrolysis include imines and alkyl halides. Fig. 2.6 showed the most common mechanism of specific acid catalyzed ester hydrolysis in an aqueous solution. The most common mechanism of specific base catalysis of ester hydrolysis is shown in Fig. 3.1.

The tetrahedral transition states formed during ester hydrolysis are very unstable and their formation is usually the rate-determining step of the reaction (Fig. 3.2).

3.1.1 Aspirin

Aspirin (acetylsalicylic acid) is an ester of an aromatic alcohol and, thus, is chemically unstable in aqueous solutions as well as in solid state in the presence of moisture. It is slightly soluble in water (3 mg/ml at 25°C) and has a melting point of about 143°C (instantaneous method), but is freely soluble in ethanol. Figure 3.3 shows the pH-rate profile for the degradation of aspirin in an aqueous solution at room temperature showing that the drug has maximum stability at a pH of about 2.5. Specific acid catalyzed hydrolysis occurs below pH 2.5 and specific base catalyzed

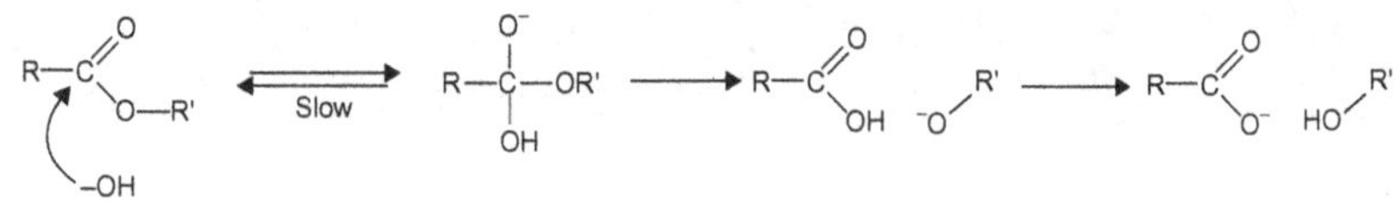

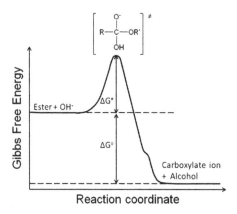

Figure 3.1 Specific base catalyzed ester hydrolysis in aqueous solution.

Figure 3.2 Reaction coordinate diagram showing the specific base catalysis of carboxylic acid ester.

hydrolysis takes over at a pH above 10, but solvent catalyzed hydrolysis occurs at pH levels between 2.5 and 10.

Possible hydrolytic pathways are displayed in Fig. 3.4. Aspirin has one ionizable group and, thus, has one unionized form and one ionized form. In theory, each form can then undergo specific acid (k_H), solvent (k_0), and specific base (k_{OH}) catalyzed hydrolysis (see Chapter 2, Section 2.8). However, it has been shown that the unionized form does not undergo specific base catalyzed hydrolysis and the ionized form does not undergo specific acid catalyzed hydrolysis:

$$-\frac{d[E]_T}{dt} = k_H[H^+][AH]+k_0[AH]+\cancel{k_{OH}[OH^-][AH]}$$
$$+\cancel{k_H'[H^+][A^-]}+k_0'[A^-]+k_{OH}'[OH^-][A^-]$$

(3.1)

The profile displayed in Fig. 3.3 can be described by Eq. 3.2:

$$-\frac{d[E]_T}{dt} = k_H[H^+][AH] + k_0[AH] + k_0'[A^-] + k_{OH}'[OH^-][A^-]$$ (3.2)

where k_H is the second-order rate constant for the specific acid catalyzed hydrolysis of the unionized aspirin (AH), k_0 is the first-order rate

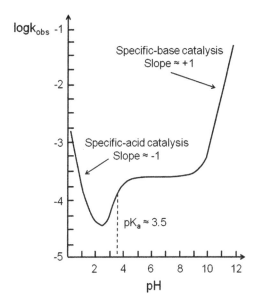

Figure 3.3 Sketch of the pH-rate profile for hydrolysis of aspirin in aqueous buffer solution at 25° C. The observed rate constant has the units of min^{-1}[1,2].

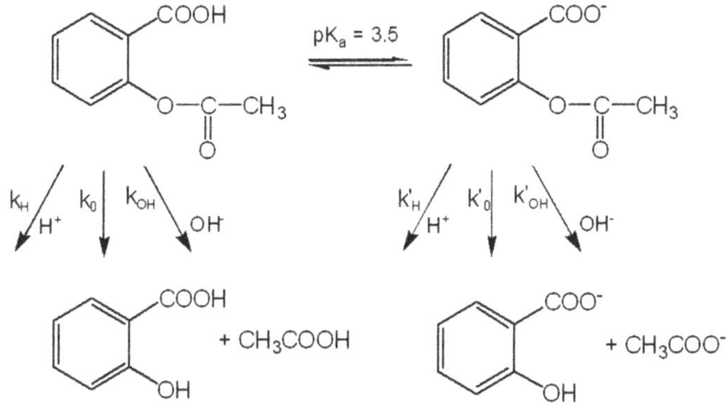

Figure 3.4 Scheme showing possible hydrolytic pathways for hydrolysis of aspirin in aqueous solution.

constant for the solvent-catalyzed (sometimes called uncatalyzed) hydrolysis of AH, k_0' is the first-order rate constant for the solvent-catalyzed hydrolysis of ionized aspirin (A$^-$), and k_{OH}' is the second-order rate constant for the specific base catalyzed hydrolysis of A$^-$. The fraction of AH and A$^-$ can be calculated from the pH and pK$_a$ values:

$$f_{AH} = \frac{[AH]}{[AH] + [A^-]} = \frac{[H^+]}{[H^+] + K_a} \tag{3.3}$$

and

$$f_{A^-} = \frac{[A^-]}{[AH] + [A^-]} = \frac{K_a}{[H^+] + K_a} \qquad (3.4)$$

Furthermore, $[AH] = f_{AH} \cdot [A]_T$, $[A^-] = f_{A^-} \cdot [A]_T$, and $[A]_T = [AH] + [A^-]$. Thus, Eq. 3.2 can be written as:

$$-\frac{d[A]_T}{dt} = (k_H[H^+]f_{AH} + k_0 f_{AH} + k_0' f_{A^-} + k_{OH}'[OH^-]f_{A^-})[A]_T \qquad (3.5)$$

where k_{obs} in Fig. 3.3 is

$$k_{obs} = k_H[H^+]f_{AH} + k_0 f_{AH} + k_0' f_{A^-} + k_{OH}'[OH^-]f_{A^-} \qquad (3.6)$$

and

$$-\frac{d[A]_T}{dt} = k_{obs}[A]_T \qquad (3.7)$$

At pH = 10 ($[H^+] \approx 10^{-10}$), Eq. 3.4 becomes:

$$f_{A^-} = \frac{K_a}{[H^+] + K_a} = \frac{10^{-3.5}}{10^{-10} + 10^{-3.5}} = 1.0 \quad \text{and thus} \quad f_{AH} = 0.0$$

At pH $\geq$ 10, Eq. 3.6 becomes $k_{obs} \approx k_{OH}'[OH^-]$. Furthermore, it can be seen that:

$$K_w = [H^+][OH^-] \quad \text{and} \quad pH = -\log[H^+]$$

$$\log[OH^-] = \log K_w - \log[H^+] = \log K_w + pH$$

$$\log k_{obs} = \log k_{OH}' + \log[OH^-] = \log k_{OH}' + \log K_w + pH$$

Thus, the theoretical slope of the linear profile ($\log k_{obs}$ versus pH) between pH 10 and pH 12 is +1.

At pH = 2 ($[H^+] \approx 10^{-2}$), Eq. 3.3 becomes:

$$f_{AH} = \frac{10^{-2}}{10^{-2} + 10^{-3.5}} = 0.97 \approx 1.0 \quad \text{and thus} \quad f_{A^-} = 0.0$$

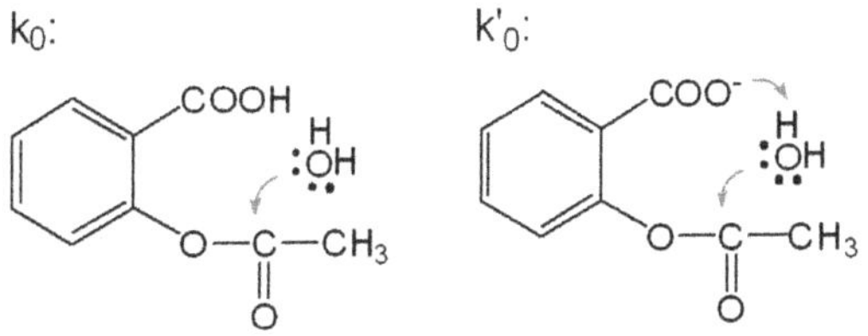

k_0: k'_0:

Figure 3.5 Solvent catalyzed hydrolysis of aspirin (nucleophilic attack of water on the ester linkage). The negative charge on the ionized aspirin "helps" the water molecule to attack the ester linkage (intramolecular catalysis).

At $pH \leq 2$, Eq. 3.6 becomes $k_{obs} = k_H[H^+]$. Furthermore, it can be seen that:

$$\log k_{obs} = \log k_H + \log [H^+] = \log k_H - pH$$

Thus, the theoretical slope of the linear profile ($\log k_{obs}$ versus pH) below pH 2 is -1.

Between pH 2 and 10 the shape of the profile is partly due to the ionization of the aspirin molecule. At the minimum ($pH \approx 2.5$) $k_H[H^+]f_{AH} \approx k_0 f_{AH}$. Then an increase in k_{obs} is observed with increasing pH with a plateau between pH 5 and 9, where $k_{obs} \approx k_0 f_{A^-} \approx k_0$. At $pH = pK_a$, $f_{AH} = f_{A^-} = 0.50$ and at $pH = 5.0$ $f_{A^-} = 1.0$. Due to intramolecular catalysis, the ionized aspirin is more unstable than the unionized form (Fig. 3.5).

When pH increases from 2.5 to 5.0, f_{AH} decreases and f_{A^-} increases and, because k'_0 is larger than k_0, k_{obs} increases. The following values were obtained at 50.8°C, ionic strength (I) 0.10 M, in a zero buffer concentration (i.e., no buffer catalysis) [1]:

$k_H = 1.32 \times 10^{-2} \, M^{-1} \, min^{-1}$
$k_0 = 1.92 \times 10^{-4} \, min^{-1}$
$k'_0 = 2.11 \times 10^{-3} \, min^{-1}$
$k_{OH} = 32.3 \, M^{-1} \, min^{-1}$

Notice that due to intramolecular catalysis, $k'_0 \approx 10 k_0$.
In general, for ester hydrolysis, $k_{OH} \gg k_H$ and, thus, esters have maximum stability at an acidic pH. There are, however, some exceptions.

Under these conditions, the following equation is obtained from Eq. 3.6:

$$k_{obs} = 1.32 \times 10^{-2}\,[H^+]f_{AH} + 1.92 \times 10^{-4}f_{AH}$$

$$+ 2.11 \times 10^{-3}f_{A^-} + 32.3[OH^-]f_{A^-}$$

This equation allows us to calculate k_{obs} (and thus the shelf-life) at any pH at 50.8°C, $I = 0.10$ M, and zero buffer concentration remembering that at 50.8°C $pK_w = 13.262$. For example, at pH 2.5, where aspirin has maximum stability, $f_{AH} = 0.91$ and $f_{A^-} = 0.09$:

$$k_{obs} = 3.80 \times 10^{-5} + 1.75 \times 10^{-4} + 1.90 \times 10^{-5} + 5.02 \times 10^{-11}$$

$$= 4.03 \times 10^{-4}\ min^{-1}$$

It can be seen that at pH 2.5, three out of four rate constants (i.e. k_H, k_0, and k'_0) contribute to k_{obs}. At pH 7.0, $I = 0.10$ M and 50.8°C $k_{obs} = 2.1 \times 10^{-3}\ min^{-1}$ and the shelf-life (t_{90}) is 0.8 h. The activation energies for the rate constants have been calculated to be 16.7 kcal/mol (69.9 kJ/mol) for k_H, 16.4 kcal/mol (68.7 kJ/mol) for k_0, 17.6 kcal/mol (73.7 kJ/mol) for k'_0, and 12.5 kcal/mol (52.3 kJ/mol) for k_{OH} [2]. With this information, we can calculate k_{obs} at various pH values and temperatures (at $I = 0.10$ M and zero buffer concentration). For example, at pH 7.0 and 25°C, $k_{obs} = 2.4 \times 10^{-4}\ min^{-1}$ and $t_{90} = 7.3$ h. Thus, aspirin is too unstable to be marketed as an aqueous solution or an aqueous suspension. On the other hand, aspirin can be found as fast dissolving effervescent tablets that contain aspirin together with sodium bicarbonate and citric acid. The tablets are dissolved in a glass of water just before intake.

In the solid state, such as in tablets, aspirin degrades in microscopic water pools (i.e., moisture) and, thus, the rate of degradation increases with increasing humidity [3,4]. Aspirin dissolves in microscopic water pools in which it is hydrolyzed to form salicylic acid and acetic acid (Fig. 3.6). The weak smell of acetic acid from solid aspirin dosage forms or pure solid aspirin indicates aspirin hydrolysis.

The water pools become saturated with aspirin and as aspirin is hydrolyzed more aspirin is dissolved. Thus, in the solid state, aspirin degradation follows pseudo zero-order kinetics (Chapter 2, Section 2.1 and Eq. 2.4):

$$-\frac{d[A]}{dt} = k_{obs}[A]_{sat} = k_{solid} \tag{3.8}$$

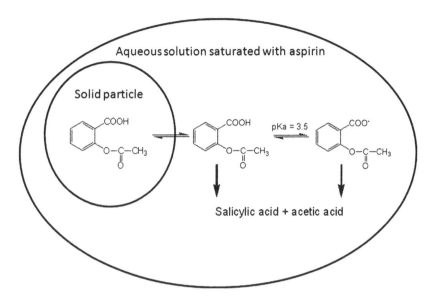

Figure 3.6 Schematic drawing of aspirin degradation in solid dosage forms in presence of moisture.

However, both the value of the observed rate constant (Eq. 3.6) and the concentration of dissolved aspirin (i.e., the fraction ionized) are pH dependent. For example, degradation of aspirin in tablets will depend on the hygroscopicity of the excipients used and the humidity (i.e., the tablets' moisture content) as well as on the pH of the microscopic aspirin solution within the tablets. The pH of pure aqueous solutions saturated with aspirin is close to 2.5, at which the drug has maximum stability. Magnesium stearate is a commonly used excipient in tablets. Magnesium stearate increases the pH of the water domains to about 4.2. This will both increase the value of k_{obs} and the amount of aspirin dissolved ($[A]_{sat}$), both of which will increase the value of k_{solid} (Eq. 3.8). Besides hydrolysis, aspirin can acetylate various drugs and excipients, such as codeine to form acetyl-codeine [5], acetaminophen (paracetamol) to form diacetylaminophen [6], and polyethylene glycols [7].

Question 3.1: The sketch in below shows the pH-rate profiles for the hydrolysis of aspirin (the solid line) and *p*-acetoxybenzoic acid (the broken line) at 25°C. Why is *p*-acetoxybenzoic acid much more stable than aspirin between pH 2 and 8?

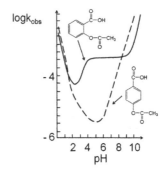

3.1.2 Procaine and Procainamide

Procaine is an ester of *p*-aminobenzoic acid. Its solubility in water is 5 mg/ml and its melting point is 61°C. Its hydrochloride is very soluble in water and has a melting point between 154°C and 158°C. Procainamide hydrochloride is also very soluble in water and has a melting point between 166°C and 170°C. Procaine and procainamide have identical structures except that in procainamide the ester linkage has been replaced by an amide linkage (Fig. 3.7) [8–10].

Based on Fig. 3.8, the equation for k_{obs} can be written as:

$$k_{obs} = k_H[H^+]f_{BH_2} + k'_H[H^+]f_{BH} + k'_0 f_{BH} + k'_{OH}[H^+]f_{BH} + k''_{OH}[OH^-]f_B$$

$$-\frac{d[B]_T}{dt} = k_{obs}[B]_T$$

$$[B]_T = [BH_2] + [BH] + [B]$$

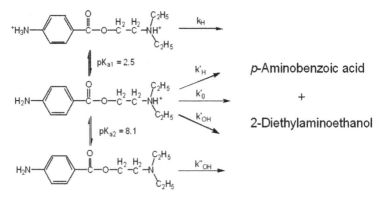

Figure 3.7 Scheme showing proposed hydrolytic pathways for hydrolysis of procaine in aqueous solution.

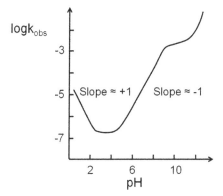

Figure 3.8 Sketch of the pH-rate profile for hydrolysis of procaine in aqueous buffer solution at 37°C. The observed rate constant has the units of min⁻¹ [9,10].

$$f_{BH_2} = \frac{[H^+]^2}{[H^+]^2 + [H^+]K_{a1} + K_{a1}K_{a2}}$$

$$f_{BH} = \frac{[H^+]K_{a1}}{[H^+]^2 + [H^+]K_{a1} + K_{a1}K_{a2}}$$

$$f_B = \frac{K_{a1}K_{a2}}{[H^+]^2 + [H^+]K_{a1} + K_{a1}K_{a2}}$$

Maximum stability is at a pH of about 3.5, at which the shelf-life of aqueous procaine solution is about 2 years at room temperature.

In procainamide, the ester linkage has been replaced by an amide linkage:

In general, amide linkages have a double binding character and, thus, are much more stable than an ester linkage:

Procainamide is much more stable in aqueous solutions than procaine. Also, in vivo procainamide in vivo procainamide is over 4 times more stable than procaine.

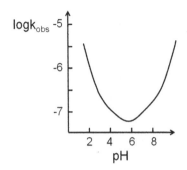

Figure 3.9 Sketch of the pH-rate profile for hydrolysis of acetaminophen in aqueous buffer solution at 25°C. The observed rate constant has the units of min^{-1} [11].

3.1.3 Acetaminophen (Paracetamol)

Acetaminophen, with a melting point between 168°C and 172°C and a pK$_a$ of about 9.7, is sparingly soluble in water (about 14 mg/ml at 25°C). The main degradation products are *p*-aminophenol and acetic acid. Its pH-rate profile displays specific acid and specific base catalysis with maximum stability at a pH of about 6 (Fig. 3.9). The shelf-life (t$_{90}$) of acetaminophen in an aqueous solution has been estimated to be over 3 years at pH 6 and 25°C [11].

3.1.4 β-Lactam Antibiotics

β-Lactam antibiotics are antibacterial agents that contain a β-lactam ring in their molecular structure, and they include penicillins, cephalosporins, monobactams, and carbapenems:

Penicillins   Cephalosporins   Monobactams   Carbapenems

The β-lactam ring is a four-member lactam ring that undergoes hydrolysis. In general, lactams are, like amides, chemically stable, but due to the structural strain of the four-member ring, the β-lactam ring is relatively rapidly hydrolyzed in aqueous solutions. The stability of the lactam ring is affected by the substituents (R). Hydrolysis of the β-lactam ring is catalyzed by intramolecular catalysis under acidic conditions:

Substituents that pull electrons away from the oxygen (i.e., electron withdrawing groups) decrease the rate of hydrolysis, while substituents that push electrons toward the oxygen (i.e., electron donating groups) enhance the rate. While ampicillin and amoxicillin are relatively stable under acidic conditions and can be given orally, benzylpenicillin is very unstable and is rapidly hydrolyzed in the stomach, which results in an extremely low oral bioavailability. *Amoxicillin* can be found in solid dosage forms (i.e., tablets and capsules), as oral suspensions, and as solutions for parenteral administration. Amoxicillin has four ionization forms and the following degradation pathway is based on the pH-rate profile (Fig. 3.10):

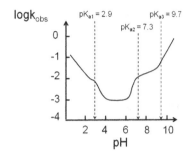

Figure 3.10 Sketch of the pH-rate profile for hydrolysis of amoxicillin in aqueous buffer solution at 35°C. The observed rate constant has the units of h^{-1} [12].

Based on Fig. 3.10, the equation for k_{obs} can be written as:

$$k_{obs} = k_H[H^+]f_{AH_3} + k'_H[H^+]f_{AH_2} + k'_0 f_{AH_2} + k'_{OH}[OH^-]f_{AH_2}$$
$$+ k''_{OH}[OH^-]f_{AH} + k'''_{OH}[OH^-]f_A$$

$$-\frac{d[A]_T}{dt} = k_{obs}[A]_T$$

$$[A]_T = [AH_3] + [AH_2] + [AH] + [A]$$

$$f_{AH_3} = \frac{[H^+]^3}{[H^+]^3 + [H^+]^2K_{a1} + [H^+]K_{a1}K_{a2} + K_{a1}K_{a2}K_{a3}}$$

$$f_{AH_2} = \frac{[H^+]^2K_{a1}}{[H^+]^3 + [H^+]^2K_{a1} + [H^+]K_{a1}K_{a2} + K_{a1}K_{a2}K_{a3}}$$

$$f_{AH} = \frac{[H^+]K_{a1}K_{a2}}{[H^+]^3 + [H^+]^2K_{a1} + [H^+]K_{a1}K_{a2} + K_{a1}K_{a2}K_{a3}}$$

$$f_A = \frac{K_{a1}K_{a2}K_{a3}}{[H^+]^3 + [H^+]^2K_{a1} + [H^+]K_{a1}K_{a2} + K_{a1}K_{a2}K_{a3}}$$

Maximum stability is at a pH of about 5, at which the shelf-life of an aqueous amoxicillin solution is less than one week at room temperature. Due to its instability, amoxicillin is marketed, not as ready-made solutions, but as a granular powder for preparation of aqueous suspensions for oral administration and as a lyophilized powder for reconstitution of a parenteral solution. Moisture in solid state formulations (e.g., tablets, capsules, and powders) promotes hydrolysis of the β-lactam ring.

Polyols (i.e., compounds with several hydroxyl groups like glucose, sucrose, dextrans, glycerol, mannitol, and sorbitol) catalyze β-lactam hydrolysis in aqueous solutions [13,14] through the formation of chemically unstable β-lactam/polyol complexes [15]. Thus, β-lactam antibiotics should not be dissolved in or mixed with carbohydrates or dissolved in, for example, isotonic glucose solutions. Likewise, metal ions such as Cu^{2+}, Zn^{2+}, and Mn^{2+}, catalyze the cleavage of the β-lactam ring through formation of complexes [16],

where k_c is much larger than k_f. For example, for benzylpenicillin and Cu^{2+}, K_c was determined to be $190\ M^{-1}$, k_f to be $0.15\ M^{-1}\ s^{-1}$, and k_c $1.2 \times 10^7\ M^{-1}\ s^{-1}$ ($k_c/k_f = 8 \times 10^7$) at 30°C. Thus, minute amounts of Cu^{2+} ions can have a significant destabilizing effect on β-lactam antibiotics.

3.1.5 Nitrogen Mustards

Nitrogen mustards are an important class of alkylating anticancer drugs that owe their activity to their ability to form reactive aziridinium ring by intramolecular displacement of the chloride by the amine nitrogen. In the presence of water, the reactive aziridinium ring (i.e., the ethylene-immonium ion) reacts with water to form inactive degradation products:

Aziridinium ring

The degradation rate is proportional to the formation of the aziridinium ring, and the presence of chloride will shift the equilibrium from the ring, thus decreasing its relative concentration and consequent mustard degradation. Protonization of the tertiary amine prevents a nucleophilic attack on the carbon to form the reactive ring. The pK_a value of nitrogen mustards is frequently about 3. At a pH below this pK_a value, nitrogen mustards are unable to form the aziridinium ring and, thus, are relatively stable.

Chlorambucil is chemically unstable in water:

Based on Fig. 3.11, the equation for k_{obs} can be written as:

$$k_{obs} = k_{H_2C}f_{H_2C} + k_{HC}f_{HC} + k_Cf_C$$

$$-\frac{d[C]_T}{dt} = k_{obs}[C]_T$$

$$[C]_T = [H_2C^+] + [HC] + [C^-]$$

$$f_{H_2C} = \frac{[H^+]^2}{[H^+]^2 + [H^+]K_{a1} + K_{a1}K_{a2}}$$

$$f_{HC} = \frac{[H^+]K_{a1}}{[H^+]^2 + [H^+]K_{a1} + K_{a1}K_{a2}}$$

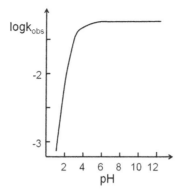

Figure 3.11 Sketch of the pH-rate profile for hydrolysis of chlorambucil in aqueous buffer solution at 40°C. The observed rate constant has the units of min^{-1} [17].

$$f_C = \frac{K_{a1}K_{a2}}{[H^+]^2 + [H^+]K_{a1} + K_{a1}K_{a2}}$$

However, since chlorambucil is essentially stable at a very acidic pH ($k_{H_2C} \approx 0$), the equation can be written as:

$$k_{obs} = \frac{k_{HC}[H^+]K_{a1} + k_C K_{a1}K_{a2}}{[H^+]^2 + [H^+]K_{a1} + K_{a1}K_{a2}}$$

3.1.6 Estramustine: How to Determine Degradation Mechanism

Estramustine sodium phosphate is a water-soluble prodrug of estramustine that is practically insoluble in water (solubility 1 µg/ml). Estramustine is a derivative of estradiol with a nitrogen mustard−carbamate ester moiety that makes it less reactive than, for example, chlorambucil. It is unable to form the reactive aziridinium ring due to the electron withdrawing properties of the carbamate ester moiety. The degradation mechanism can be revealed by determining the degradation rate under various experimental conditions.

Estramustine sodium phosphate   Estramustine   Estradiol

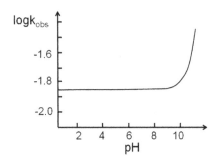

Figure 3.12 Sketch of the pH-rate profile for hydrolysis of estramustine in aqueous buffer solution at 80° C. The observed rate constant has the units of min⁻¹[16].

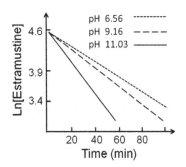

Figure 3.13 First-order plots (ln[drug] versus time plots) for the degradation of estramustine in aqueous solution at 80° C.

The degradation of estramustine was studied in aqueous solutions [18]. The pH-rate profile (Fig. 3.12) is very different from other nitrogen mustards, such as that of chlorambucil (Fig. 3.11), indicating that hydrolysis of this nitrogen mustard drug proceeds through a different mechanism.

Estramustine does not display any pK_a values in the pH range from 1 to 11. Based on Fig. 3.12, the rate equation for the disappearance of estramustine in aqueous solutions is:

$$k_{obs} = k_0 + k_{OH}[OH^-] \qquad -\frac{d[\text{Estramustine}]_T}{dt} = k_{obs}[\text{Estramustine}]$$

A liquid chromatographic method was used to monitor the disappearance of estramustine as a function of time (Fig. 3.13). The method showed the appearance of a degradation product later identified as estradiol (Fig. 3.14).

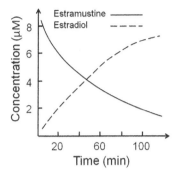

Figure 3.14 The disappearance of estramustine and appearance of estradiol in aqueous phosphate buffer solution at pH 7.5 and 80° C.

Table 3.1 The Observed First-Order Rate Constants (K_{obs}) for the Degradation of Estramustine in Aqueous Phosphate Buffer Solution at pH 7.5 and Various Temperatures.

Temperature		k_{obs} (min^{-1})
(°C)	(K)	
86	359	260×10^{-4}
80	353	154×10^{-4}
75	348	94.8×10^{-4}
70	343	62.3×10^{-4}
Calculated values:		
25	298	4.62×10^{-4}
5	278	0.03×10^{-4}

Figure 3.13 shows that the estramustine degradation follows the first-order rate equation (see Chapter 2, Eq. 2.15), while Fig. 3.14 shows that the rate of estradiol appearance is equal to the rate of estramustine disappearance. Then the effect of temperature (Table 3.1) and the dielectric constant (Table 3.2) on the degradation rate was investigated.

Plotting $\ln \frac{k}{T}$ versus $\frac{1}{T}$ according to Eq. 2.130, gives us a straight line from which the enthalpy of activation ($\Delta H^{\neq}$) is calculated from the slope, and the entropy of activation ($\Delta S^{\neq}$) is calculated from the intercept (see Chapter 2, Fig. 2.10). From the values given in Table 3.1, $\Delta H^{\neq}$ was

Table 3.2 The Effect of Dielectric Constant (E) on the Observed First-Order Rate Constant (K_{obs}) in Aqueous Phosphate Buffer Solution at pH 7.4 and 80 C

Dioxane (% v/v)	ε^a	k_{obs} (min^{-1})
0	60.55	1.478×10^{-2}
10	53.08	1.273×10^{-2}
20	45.77	0.933×10^{-2}
30	38.64	0.619×10^{-2}
^{a}Calculated at 80° C [19].		

determined to be 89.3 kJ mol^{-1} (21.4 k cal mol^{-1}) and $\Delta S^{\neq}$ to be -62.0 J mol^{-1} K^{-1}(-14.8 cal mol^{-1} K^{-1}). This rather large $\Delta H^{\neq}$ and low negative $\Delta S^{\neq}$ could indicate a unimolecular reaction (i.e., only one molecule in the rate-determining step (RDS)). Equation 2.130 can also be used to calculate k_{obs} at 25 and 5°C (pH of 7.5), and from the rate constants, the shelf-life (t_{90}) can be estimated (Eq. 2.19) to be about 6.7 h at 25°C and about 24 days at 5°C. Table 3.2 shows that k_{obs} decreases with a decreasing ε, suggesting some charge development in the transition state.

The value of k_{obs} was also determined for deuterium oxide (D$_2$O) at pH 6.5 and 80°C, and the isotope effect was determined:

$$\text{Isotope effect} = \frac{k_{H_2O}}{k_{D_2O}} = \frac{1.35 \times 10^{-2} \text{ min}^{-1}}{1.23 \times 10^{-2} \text{ min}^{-1}} = 1.10$$

This small isotope effect is probably not due to the cleavage of an O$-$H bond, but rather due to some secondary effects. This is consistent with unimolecular RDS. Finally, the addition of chloride ions (Cl$^-$) to the reaction media did not affect the k_{obs} value, indicating that Cl$^-$ is not released during the RDS. These observations agree with the following degradation mechanism:

Transition state

Knowing the degradation mechanism of a given drug can help the pharmaceutical scientist to design stable formulations containing the drug.

Question 3.2: The figure below shows how the half-life ($t_{1/2}$) for chlorambucil hydrolysis increases with increasing chloride (Cl^-) concentration [20]. Why does the $t_{1/2}$ increase with increasing $[Cl^-]$?

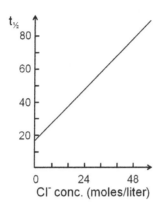

3.2 OXIDATION

Oxidative reactions are somewhat common drug degradation pathways. Most drugs exist in their reduced form and oxygen, which participates in most oxidation reactions, is abundant in the environment (e.g., 20.95% of the atmosphere). Fresh water in an open vial contains about 6 ml/liter of O_2 at 25°C, and about twice as much at 0°C. As in the case of hydrolytic reactions, the rate of oxidation is both pH- and temperature-dependent, and as in the case of hydrolysis, oxidative reactions are much faster in aqueous solutions than in the solid state. In addition, metal ions and light can have catalytic effects on oxidative reactions.

Oxidation is a loss of electrons or an increase in the oxidation state and reduction is a gain in electrons or a decrease in the oxidation state. Redox reaction is an electron transfer process:

$$Reduced\ form \rightleftharpoons Oxidized\ form + ne^-$$

where the reduced form loses n number of electrons (e^-). A simple oxidation is the oxidation of methanol (CH_3OH) to form formaldehyde (CH_2O), formic acid ($CHOOH$), or carbon dioxide (CO_2). A simple reduction can, for example, be hydrogenation of carbon−carbon double bonds. In comparison to hydrolysis, the oxidative degradation pathways are, in general, rather complex.

3.2.1 Morphine

In its unionized form, morphine is almost insoluble in water (solubility is about 0.2 mg/ml) but it is most often used in a salt form such as morphine hydrochloride (solubility is about 40 mg/ml at room temperature). Morphine has two pK_a values: $pK_{a1} = 8.0$ (protonated amino group) and $pK_{a2} = 9.9$ (phenol) at room temperature. The oxidative degradation pathway of morphine is rather complex in which the phenol group and the amino group play important roles [21]. Below are some examples of degradation products:

The oxidative degradation kinetics are frequently rather complex, depending on the oxygen concentration as well as other external factors, such as pH, temperature, and buffer salts. In aqueous solutions saturated with oxygen (i.e., $[O_2]$ = constant), the rate constants for morphine degradation are:

$$k_{HM} = k'_{HM}[O_2]$$

$$k_M = k'_M[O_2]$$

When only the protonation of the amino group is considered, then the equation for k_{obs} is (for pH levels from 2 to 7):

$$k_{obs} = k_{HM}\frac{[H^+]}{[H^+] + K_{a1}} + k_M \frac{K_{a1}}{[H^+] + K_{a1}} = k_{HM}f_{HM} + k_M f_M$$

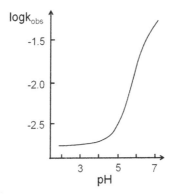

Figure 3.15 Sketch of the pH-rate profile for oxidation of morphine in aqueous solution at 95°C and in the presence of excess oxygen. The observed rate constant has the units of h^{-1} [20].

Figure 3.15 shows the effect of pH on k_{obs}. At 95°C, pK_{a1} was determined to be 6.77, k_{HM} to be $1.77 \times 10^{-3}\,h^{-1}$, and k_M to be $8.03 \times 10^{-2}\,h^{-1}$. E_a was estimated to be 22.8 kcal/mol at a pH between 5.0 and 6.5 [22].

3.2.2 Ascorbic Acid

L-Ascorbic acid (vitamin C) is a water-soluble compound frequently used as an antioxidant in food products due to its mild reducing properties. Ascorbic acid has two pK_a values: $pK_{a1} = 4.2$ and $pK_{a2} = 11.6$ at room temperature.

HO— ... O ...O pK_{a1} HO— ... O ...O   ⟷   HO— ... O ...O⁻
HO H̄ ... ... HO H̄ ... HO H̄
HO   OH   ⁻O   OH   O   OH

L-Ascorbic acid (AH₂)   Ascorbate (AH⁻)

The rate of oxidative degradation of ascorbic acid is at its maximum at the pK_a value at which $[AH_2] = [AH^-]$, suggesting the following degradation mechanism [23]:

$$AH_2 + O_2 \xrightarrow{k_1} \text{Product}$$
$$AH_2/AH^- + O_2 \xrightarrow{k_2} \text{Product}$$
$$AH^- + O_2 \xrightarrow{k_3} \text{Product}$$

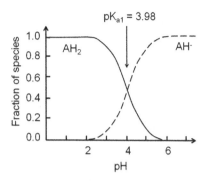

Figure 3.16 Fraction of AH_2 (unbroken curve) and AH^- (broken curve) as a function of pH at 67°C [21].

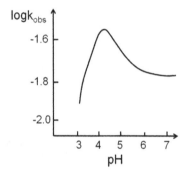

Figure 3.17 Sketch of the pH-rate profile for oxidation of ascorbic acid in aqueous solution under aerobic conditions at 67°C. The observed rate constant has the units of h^{-1} [21].

where k_2 is much larger than k_1 and k_3. Ascorbic acid is available both in solid dosage forms (e.g., tablets) and in aqueous parenteral solutions. Ascorbic acid degrades in the solid state with discoloration under the influence of moisture [24]. Both moisture and air accelerate ascorbic acid degradation in the solid state.

3.2.3 Autoxidation

Autoxidation (auto-oxidation) is a complex oxidation mechanism that proceeds through a free radical chain process. It is a common degradation mechanism for unsaturated fats, but a number of drugs containing carbon−carbon double bonds also undergo autoxidation. In general, the free radical chain process consists of three steps [25]:

Initiation $RH \rightarrow R^\bullet + H^\bullet$

Propagation $\begin{cases} R^\bullet + O_2 \rightarrow ROO^\bullet \\ ROO^\bullet + RH \underset{RDS}{\rightarrow} ROOH + R^\bullet \end{cases}$

Termination $\begin{cases} ROO^\bullet + ROO^\bullet \rightarrow \text{Non-radical products} \\ ROO^\bullet + ROOH \rightarrow \text{Non-radical products} \end{cases}$

A free radical is formed in the initiation step, frequently through the thermal or photochemical hemolytic cleavage of an R−H bond. The initiation is catalyzed by metal ions such as Cu^{2+}, Ni^{2+}, and Fe^{3+}. Molecular oxygen is added to the free radical in the propagation step and then in the rate-determining step (RDS), the peroxyl radical extracts the hydrogen atom from RH to form another $R^\bullet$ radical. The rate of the RDS depends mainly on the strength of the C−H bond that is being cleaved. In the termination step, the chain reaction is broken when two free radicals react to form nonradical products. The rancidification of fat, which gives a distinct rancid smell (due to the formation of volatile aldehydes and ketones), is an example of autoxidation:

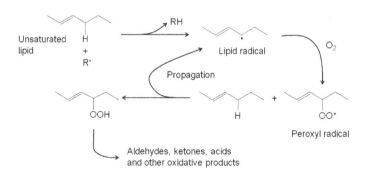

3.2.4 Retinol

Retinol (all-*trans*-retinol; vitamin A_1) is insoluble in water (solubility is about 0.04 mg/ml at room temperature). Retinol is a polyunsaturated compound and as such is susceptible to oxidative degradation as well as to cis−trans isomerization.

| Retinol | Tretinoin | Isotretinoin |

Related drugs are all-*trans*-retinoic acid (tretinoin) and 13-*cis*-retinoic acid (isotretinoin). Retinol, tretinoin, and isotretinoin are polyunsaturated compounds with numerous C−C double bonds and are, as such, subject to autoxidation. Retinyl palmitate (the ester of retinol and palmitic acid) is less susceptible to autoxidation than the free retinol and, thus, is used in aqueous parenteral and oral solutions [26].

3.2.5 Antioxidants

Antioxidants are pharmaceutical excipients that prevent or delay oxidative degradation of active ingredients. Antioxidants are classified into three groups: phenolic antioxidants (sometimes called true antioxidants), reducing agents, and chelating agents (Table 3.3).

Phenolic antioxidants are sterically hindered phenols that react with free radicals, blocking the chain reaction.

| BHT | Propyl gallate | BHA |

Table 3.3 Classes and Examples of Antioxidants

Phenolic Antioxidants	Reducing Agents	Chelating Agents
Butylated hydroxyanisole (BHA)	Ascorbic acid	Citric acid
Butylated hydroxytoluene (BHT)	Ascorbyl palmitate	Disodium edetate
tetra-Butylhydroquinone	Monothioglycerol	Fumaric acid
Gallic acid	Sodium bisulfite	Malic acid
Propyl gallate	Sodium metabisulfite	Phosphoric acid
α-Tocopherol	Sodium sulfite	Tartaric acid

These hindered phenols are radical-trapping antioxidants for oxy- and peroxy radicals. The phenoxy radicals formed with their bulky substituents are stabilized by steric hindrance and cannot attach drugs or unsaturated fatty acids to maintain the chain reaction (propagation step), for example BHT:

The radical formed is stabilized by delocalization of the unpaired electron around the phenol ring to form a stable resonance hybrid (i.e. low-energy radical):

BHT, propyl gallate, and BHA are examples of synthetic hindered phenols. An example of a natural hindered phenol is α-tocopherol.

Reducing agents are compounds that have lower redox potentials and, thus, are more readily oxidized than the drug they are intended to protect. Reducing agents scavenge oxygen from the medium and, thus, delay or prevent drug oxidation.

Chelating agents are sometimes called antioxidant synergists. Metal ions, such as Co^{2+}, Cu^{2+}, Fe^{3+}, Fe^{2+}, and Mn^{2+}, shorten the induction period and increase the oxidation rate. Trace amounts of these metal ions are frequently introduced to drug products during manufacturing. Chelating agents do not possess antioxidant activity as such, but enhance the action of phenolic antioxidants by reacting with catalyzing metal ions to make them inactive.

Antioxidant synergism is the cooperative effect of antioxidants, or an antioxidant with other compounds, to produce better antioxidant activity than the sum of activities of the individual antioxidants when used by themselves. For example, two or more phenolic antioxidants can give synergistic effects due to differences in steric hindrance. Phenolic antioxidants are used in combination with chelating agents because the chelating agents decrease the oxidation rates by inhibiting metal-catalyzed oxidation, resulting in the formation of fewer free radicals.

A commercial vitamin A solution contains 50,000 International Units of retinyl palmitate in 1.00 ml of an aqueous vehicle consisting of 12% polysorbate 80 (solubilizer), 0.5% chlorobutanol (antibacterial and antifungal agent), 0.1% citric acid (chelating agent), and 0.03% BHA and 0.03% BHT (phenolic antioxidants). The pH is adjusted to 6.8 with sodium hydroxide. In this formulation BHA, BHT, and citric acid have a synergistic antioxidant effect.

Question 3.3: The sketch below shows the effect of various additives on the rate of disappearance of COL-3 (a chemically modified tetracycline) from an aqueous pH 10.3 phosphate buffer at 25°C in the presence of light [27]. The concentration of the additives was in all cases 0.005% (w/v). Why do the additives increase the stability of COL-3?

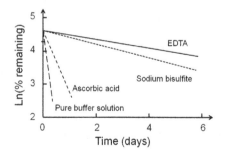

3.3 ISOMERIZATION

Isomerization is a degradation process in which a drug degrades to form a product with an identical chemical formula (i.e., isomers). Isomers have the same chemical composition but a different configuration or structure and possess different physicochemical properties. Most drug receptors and many enzymes are stereoselective and stereospecific; thus, drug isomers will have different biological properties, including pharmacological and toxicological properties. For example, the natural L-ascorbic acid has antiscorbutic activity, but the synthetic D-ascorbic acid does not. Both, however, have antioxidant properties. There are two main categories of isomers (i.e., stereoisomers and structural isomers).

3.3.1 Stereoisomers

Ephedrine has two chiral centers (n = 2), giving rise to four stereoisomers ($n^2 = 4$). All four stereoisomers are known compounds with known biological properties:

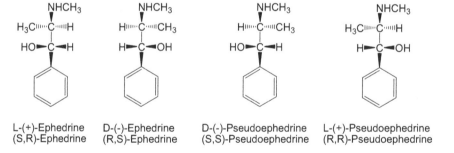

L-(+)-Ephedrine   D-(-)-Ephedrine   D-(-)-Pseudoephedrine   L-(+)-Pseudoephedrine
(S,R)-Ephedrine   (R,S)-Ephedrine   (S,S)-Pseudoephedrine   (R,R)-Pseudoephedrine

   L-(+)-Ephedrine and D-(−)-ephedrine are *enantiomers* (or mirror images of each other) and so are D-(−) pseudoephedrine and L-(+)-pseudoephedrine. L-(+)-Ephedrine and D-(−) pseudoephedrine are *diastereomers*. Diastereomers occur when compounds have two or more chiral centers and different configurations at one or more, but not all, of the centers (i.e., not mirror images of each other). *Racemization* refers to the conversion of a pure enantiomer into a mixture in which two (or more) enantiomers are present. *Racemate* is a mixture containing equal amounts of the enantiomers. Epimers are diastereomers that differ in configuration at only one chiral center.

| Tetracycline | 4-*epi*-Tetracycline |

Cis/trans isomers (also called *geometric isomers* or *E/Z isomers*) are a form of stereoisomers describing the orientation of functional groups within a molecule, usually around double bonds:

cis or Z isomer   trans or E isomer

3.3.2 Structural Isomers

Structural isomers (constitutional isomers) have the same molecular formula, but the atoms are arranged in a different way. For example, *n*-propanol (propan-1-ol) and isopropanol (propan-2-ol) are structural isomers with the same molecular formula (C_3H_8O) but different physicochemical properties, like boiling point and density. Propanol and isopropanol are *position isomers*. *Tautomers* are also structural isomers but they are readily interconverted by a chemical reaction called tautomerization.

3.3.3 Epinephrine

L-(−)-Epinephrine (*l*-adrenaline or 4-[(1R)-1-hydroxy-2-(methylamino) ethyl]benzene-1,2-diol) has one chiral center.

In aqueous solutions, epinephrine undergoes specific acid catalyzed racemization [28].

However, the main degradation route of epinephrine under aerobic conditions is oxidation to form adrenochrome (the solution goes from colorless to pink) and other oxidation products. The rate of oxidation increases with increasing pH, while the rate of racemization decreases with increasing pH. The optimum stability of the aqueous epinephrine solutions has been estimated to be between pH 3.0 and 3.8, at which the total rate of degradation (i.e., the rate of racemization and the rate of oxidation) is at its minimum [29].

3.3.4 Tetracyclines

Tetracycline   Doxycycline   Oxytetracycline

Tetracyclines form a group of naturally occurring antibiotics consisting of four hydrocarbon rings. The rings are lettered from A to D, and the numbers begin at the bottom of ring A. Tetracyclines are fairly stable in aqueous solutions under acidic conditions, but are somewhat labile under basic conditions. However, under neutral to acidic conditions, tetracycline and other tetracyclines undergo epimerization [30].

Tetracyclines do also form several tautomeric forms, for example:

Tetracycline has three pKa values. $pKa_1 = 3.3$ (tautomeric stabilization of the anion formed):

$pKa_2 = 7.3$ (tautomeric stabilization of the anion formed):

$pKa_3 = 9.1$:

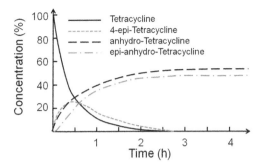

Figure 3.18 Sketch of the concentration profile of the degradation products of tetracycline in aqueous solution at pH 1.5 and 75°C [31].

In acidic solutions, tetracyclines undergo epimerization and dehydration (Fig. 3.18):

Tetracycline

4-epi-Tetracycline

anhydro-Tetracycline

epi-anhydro-Tetracycline

In alkaline solutions, the enolone moiety in position 11−12 is attacked by hydroxyl ions:

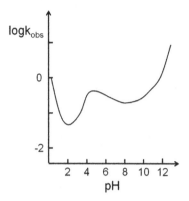

Figure 3.19 Sketch of the pH-rate profile for the degradation of oxytetracycline in aqueous solution at 60° C (I = 0.5). The observed rate constant has the units of h^{-1} [32].

The pH-rate profile of oxytetracycline at 60°C, at zero buffer concentration, and at ionic strength 0.5 is shown in Fig. 3.19 [32]. The three pKa values of oxytetracycline are 3.3, 7.3, and 9.1 at 25°C and, thus, the drug exists in four ionization forms:

$$H_3O^+ \xrightleftharpoons{pKa_1} H_2O^{+-} \xrightleftharpoons{pKa_2} HO^{+2-} \xrightleftharpoons{pKa_3} O^{2-}$$

with rate constants k_H, k_0, k_0', k_0'', k_0''', k_{OH}'''.

Based on Fig. 3.19, the equation for k_{obs} can be written as:

$$k_{obs} = k_H[H^+]f_{H_3O} + k_0 f_{H_3O} + k_0' f_{H_2O} + k_0'' f_{HO} + k_0''' f_O + k_{OH}'''[OH^-]f_O$$

$$-\frac{d[O]_T}{dt} = k_{obs}[O]_T$$

$$[O]_T = [H_3O^+] + [H_2O^{+-}] + [HO^{+2-}] + [O^{2-}]$$

$$f_{H_3O} = \frac{[H^+]^3}{[H^+]^3 + [H^+]^2 K_{a1} + [H^+]K_{a1}K_{a2} + K_{a1}K_{a2}K_{a3}} \quad \text{and so on.}$$

The values of the rate constants for the pH-rate profile shown in Fig. 3.19 were determined at 60°C and I = 0.5 [32]:

$k_H = 1.7 \ M^{-1} \ h^{-1}$
$k_0 = 0.03 \ h^{-1}$
$k_0' = 0.42 \ h^{-1}$
$k_0'' = 0.22 \ h^{-1}$
$k_0''' = 0.30 \ h^{-1}$
$k_{OH}''' = 43.4 \ M^{-1} \ h^{-1}$

Oxytetracycline has maximum stability at a pH of about 2.

3.3.5 Pilocarpine

Pilocarpine (pKa = 7.1 at 25°C) is an antiglaucoma drug administered as aqueous eye drop solutions. Pilocarpine is a lactone with two asymmetric carbon atoms that undergoes hydrolysis under both acidic and alkaline conditions. Under alkaline conditions, epimerization is a minor degradation pathway ($\sim 20\%$):

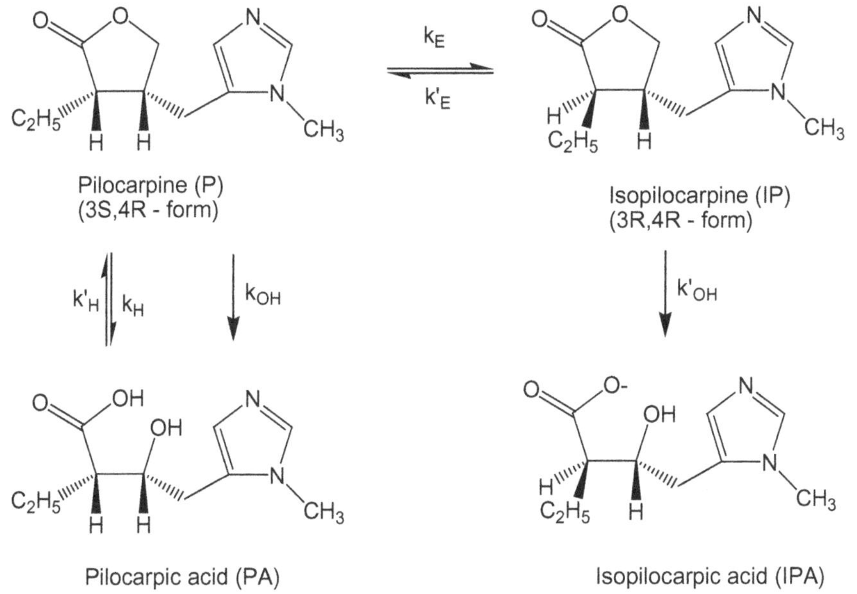

Pilocarpine (P)
(3S,4R - form)

Isopilocarpine (IP)
(3R,4R - form)

Pilocarpic acid (PA)

Isopilocarpic acid (IPA)

The mechanism of pilocarpine epimerization in alkaline solution is as follows:

The rate equation can be written as (disregarding the ionization of pilocarpine):

$$-\frac{d[P]}{dt} = k_H[P]\left[H^+\right] + k_{OH}[P][OH^-] + k_E[P][OH^-]$$
$$- k'_H[PA]\left[H^+\right] - k'_E[IP][OH^-]$$

In aqueous solutions, pilocarpine has maximum stability at a pH of about 5 at which the shelf-life is greater than 5 years at 25°C.

3.3.6 Cis–Trans Isomerization

Cis–trans isomerization is also called geometrical isomerization, which describes the relative orientation of functional groups within a molecule that, in general, contain double bonds. Cis–trans isomerization, however, is also known in ring structures in which the rotation of bonds is restricted. An example of cis–trans isomerization is the degradation of retinol (all-trans vitamin A_1):

Related drugs, such as all-trans-retinoic acid (tretinoin), 9-cis-retinoic acid (alitretinoin) and 13-cis-retinoic acid (isotretinoin), are also susceptible to cis−trans isomerization. However, oxidation is most often the main degradation pathway of retinol and related compounds.

3.4 PHOTOCHEMICAL DEGRADATION

Numerous drugs can undergo photochemical decomposition, some more readily than others, and in most cases the reaction mechanism is rather complex. For example, piroxicam degrades via two pathways: a hydrolytic pathway and a photochemical pathway [33]:

The degradation pathway of piroxicam and the relative concentrations of the products formed depend on the conditions, including the pH of the medium. Other common photochemical degradation pathways include dehalogenation (e.g., norfloxacin, ciprofloxacin, and chlorpromazine), decarboxylation (e.g., ibuprofen and naproxen) and rearrangement (e.g., diazepam, metronidazole, and diethylstilbestrol).

3.5 DECARBOXYLATION

Decarboxylation does not have to be a photochemical degradation. For example, decarboxylation of p-aminosalicylic acid has been shown to be a rate-controlling proton addition followed by rapid decarboxylation [34].

The value of the rate constant at a pH between 1 and 7 depends on the relative concentration of the zwitterion ($pKa_1 = 1.8$; $pKa_2 = 3.6$):

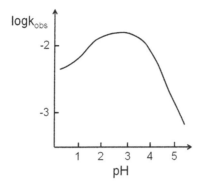

Figure 3.20 Sketch of the pH-rate profile for the decarboxylation of p-aminosalicylic acid in aqueous solution at 25°C (I = 0.5). The observed rate constant has the units of h⁻¹ [34].

$$k_{obs} = k_{AH_2}[H^+]f_{AH_2} + k_{AH^\pm}[H^+]f_{AH^\pm} \text{ where } k_{AH^\pm} \approx 100k_{AH_2}$$

Maximum degradation is observed at the isoelectric point (pH = 2.7) at which k_{obs} has maximum value (Fig. 3.20). *p*-Aminosalicylic acid has maximum stability at a pH between 9 and 10.

3.6 DEHYDRATION

Prostaglandin E_2 (pKa = 5.0) dehydrates readily in aqueous solutions to form prostaglandins A_2 and B_2 [35,36].

Prostaglandin E_2 Prostaglandin A_2 Prostaglandin B_2

The pH-rate profile (Fig. 3.21) displays specific acid- and specific base-catalysis:

$$k_{obs} = k_H[H^+]f_{PH} + k_0 f_{PH} + k'_0 f_P + k'_{OH}[OH^-]f_P$$

where k_H is the rate constant for the specific acid catalyzed dehydration of unionized prostaglandin E_2 (PH), k_0 is the solvent catalyzed (or uncatalyzed) dehydration of PH, k'_0 is the solvent catalyzed dehydration of the

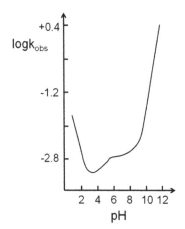

+0.4

$logk_{obs}$

-1.2

-2.8

2 4 6 8 10 12
ph

Figure 3.21 Sketch of the pH-rate profile for the dehydration of prostaglandin E_2 in aqueous 5% (v/v) ethanol solution at 25°C. The observed rate constant has the units of h^{-1} [33].

ionized prostaglandin E_2 (P), and k'_{OH} is the specific base catalyzed dehydration of P. Various other drugs have a tendency to undergo dehydration as a form of degradation, such as erythromycin and streptovitacin A.

Question 3.4: The following figure shows the reaction profile for prostaglandin E_2 (PGE$_2$) at pH 8.0 and 60°C [35]. Why is prostaglandin B$_2$ more stable than prostaglandin A$_2$? What type of a reaction is prostaglandin $A_2 \rightarrow$ prostaglandin B$_2$?

Prostaglandin E$_2$

Prostaglandin A$_2$

Prostaglandin B$_2$

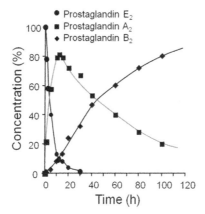

3.7 POLYMERIZATION

Formaldehyde is a gas, but forms a hydrate, methanediol ($H_2C(OH)_2$), in aqueous solutions:

$$CH_2O + H_2O \rightleftharpoons HO-CH_2-OH$$
$$\text{Methanediol}$$

Methanediol is chemically reactive and reacts with itself to form polymers:

$$HO-CH_2-OH + HO-CH_2-OH \rightarrow HO-CH_2-O-CH_2-OH$$

$$\rightarrow \rightarrow \rightarrow HO-[CH_2-O]_n-CH_2-OH$$

An aqueous formaldehyde solution, known as formalin, contains 40% (v/v) formaldehyde, most of which exists as water-soluble polymers ($n \leq 7$). Larger polymers ($n > 7$) are less water-soluble, and the precipitate is known as paraformaldehyde. Methanol is frequently added to aqueous formaldehyde solutions to prevent formation of a white paraformaldehyde precipitation. The water-soluble cyclic formaldehyde trimer, known as 1,3,5-trioxane (($CH_2O)_3$), also formed in aqueous formaldehyde solutions.

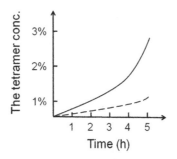

Figure 3.22 Sketch of the rate of the penicillin tetramer formation in aqueous ampicillin solution at pH 6 and 22°C. The initial ampicillin concentration was 10% (w/v) (the broken curve) and 20% (w/v) (the solid curve).

Some β-lactam antibiotics, such as ampicillin, are also known to form polymers [37].

Question 3.5: How does methanol stabilize aqueous formaldehyde solutions?

Why did the investigator monitor formation of the penicillin tetramer instead of the polymer?

Why do the formation curves shown in Fig. 3.22 display positive deviation from linearity?

REFERENCES

[1] T. Loftsson, N. Bodor, Improved delivery through biological membranes IX: kinetics and mechanism of hydrolysis of methylsulfinylmethyl 2-acetoxybenzoate and related aspirin prodrugs, J. Pharm. Sci. 70 (1981) 750–755.

[2] E.R. Garrett, The kinetics of solvolysis of acyl esters of salicylic acid, J. Am. Chem. Soc. 79 (1957) 3401–3408.

[3] L.J. Leeson, A.M. Mattocks, Decomposition of aspirin in the solid state, J. Pharm. Sci. 47 (1958) 329–333.

[4] J.T. Carstensen, F. Attarchi, X.-P. Hou, Decomposition of aspirin in the solid state in the presence of limited amounts of moisture, J. Pharm. Sci. 74 (1985) 741–745.

[5] A.L. Jacobs, A.E. Dilatush, S. Weinstein, J.J. Windheuser, Formation of acetylcodeine from aspirin and codeine, J. Pharm. Sci. 55 (1966) 893–895.

[6] K.T. Koshy, A.E. Troup, R.N. Duvall, R.C. Conwell, L.L. Shankle, Acetylation of acetaminophen in tablet formulations containing aspirin, J. Pharm. Sci. 56 (1967) 1117–1121.

[7] H.W. Jun, C.W. Whitworth, L.A. Luzzi, Decomposition of aspirin in polyethylene glycols, J. Pharm. Sci. 61 (1972) 1160–1162.

[8] K. Bullock, J.S. Cannell, The preparation of solutions of procaine and adrenaline hydrochlorides for surgical use, Quart. J. Pharm. Pharmacol. 14 (1941) 241–251.

[9] T. Higuchi, A. Havinga, L.W. Busse, The kinetics of the hydrolysis of procaine, J. Pharm. Sci., Ed. 39 (1950) 405–410.

[10] K.A. Connors, G.L. Amidon, V.J. Stella, Chemical Stability of Pharmaceuticals. A handbook for pharmacists, John Wiley & Sons, New York, 1986.

[11] K.T. Koshy, J.L. Lach, Stability of aqueous solutions of N-acetyl-p-aminophenol, J. Pharm. Sci. 50 (1961) 113–118.

[12] H. Zia, N. Shalchian, F. Borhanian, Kinetics of amoxycillin degradation in aqueous solutions, Can. J. Pharm. Sci. 12 (1977) 80–83.

[13] H. Bundgaard, C. Larsen, Kinetics and mechanism of the sucrose-accelerated degradation of penicillins in aqueous solutions, Int. J. Pharm. 1 (1978) 95–104.

[14] H. Bundgaard, C. Larsen, The influence of carbohydrates and polyhydric alcohols on the stability of cephalosporins in aqueous solutions, Int. J. Pharm. 16 (1983) 319–325.

[15] T. Loftsson, B.J. Ólafsdóttir, Cyclodextrin-accelerated degradation of β-lactam antibiotics in aqueous solutions, Int. J. Pharm. 67 (1991) R5–R7.

[16] R. Méndez, T. Alemany, J. Martín-Villacorta, Catalysis of hydrolysis and aminolysis of non-classical antibiotics by metal ions and metal chelates, Chem. Pharm. Bull. 40 (1992) 3228–3233.

[17] T. Loftsson, S. Björnsdóttir, G. Pálsdóttir, N. Bodor, The effects of 2-hydroxypropyl-b-cyclodextrin on the solubility and stability of chlorambucil and melphalan in aqueous solution, Int. J. Pharm. 57 (1989) 63–72.

[18] T. Loftsson, B.J. Olafsdottir, J. Baldvinsdottir, Estramustine: hydrolysis, solubilization, and stabilization in aqueous solutions, Int. J. Pharm. 79 (1992) 107–112.

[19] B.B. Owen, H.D. Harris, The physical chemistry of electrolytic solutions, Reinhold, New York, 1958.

[20] D.C. Chatterji, R.L. Yeager, J.F. Gallelli, Kinetics of chlorambucil hydrolysis using high-pressure liquid chromatography, J. Pharm. Sci. 71 (1982) 50–54.

[21] A. Vermeire, J.P. Remon, Stability and compatibility of morphine, Int. J. Pharm. 187 (1999) 17–51.

[22] S.Y. Yeh, J. Lach, Stability of morphine in aqueous solutions. III. Kinetics of morphine degradation in aqueous solutions, J. Pharm. Sci. 50 (1961) 35–42.

[23] S.M. Blaug, B. Hajratwala, Kinetics of aerobic oxidation of ascorbic acid, J. Pharm. Sci. 61 (1972) 556–562.

[24] A.B. Shephard, S.C. Nichols, A. Braithwaite, Moisture induced solid phase degradation of L-ascorbic acid. Part 1: a kinetic study using tristimulus colorimetry and a quantitative HPLC assay, Talanta 48 (1999) 585–593.

[25] N.A. Porter, S.E. Caldwell, K.A. Mills, Mechanism of free radical oxidation of unstaturated lipids, Lipids 30 (1995) 277–290.

[26] M.E. Carlotti, V. Rossatto, M. Gallarate, Vitamin A and vitamin A palmitate stability over time and under UVA and UVB radiation, Int. J. Pharm. 240 (2002) 85–94.

[27] S. Pinsuwan, F.A. Alvarez-Núñez, E.S. Tabibi, S.H. Yalkowsky, Degradation kinetics of 4-dedimethylamino sancycline, a new anti-tumor agent, in aqueous solutions, Int. J. Pharm. 181 (1999) 31–40.

[28] L.C. Schroeter, T. Higuchi, A kinetic study of acid-catalyzed racemization of epinephrine, J. Am. Pharm. Assoc. Sci. Ed. 47 (1958) 426–430.

[29] P.C.M. Hoevenaars, Stabiliteit van adrenaline in injectievloeistoffen, Pharm. Weekbl. 100 (1965) 1151–1162.

[30] B. Halling-Sørensen, G. Sengeløv, J. Tjørnelund, Toxicity of tetracyclines and tetracycline degradation products to environmentally relevant bacteria, including selected tetracycline-resistant bacteria, Arch. Environ. Contam. Toxicol. 42 (2002) 263–271.

[31] P.H. Yuen, T.D. Sokoloski, Kinetics of concomitant degradation of tetracycline to epitetracycline, anhydrotetracycline, and epianhydrotetracycline in acid phosphate soution, J. Pharm. Sci. 66 (1977) 1648–1650.

[32] B. Vej-Hansen, H. Bundgaard, B. Kreilgård, Kinetic degradation of oxytetracycline in aqueous solution, Arch. Pharma. Chem. Sci. Ed. 6 (1978) 151–163.

[33] D.T. Modhave, T. Handa, R.P. Shah, S. Sing, Successful charaterization of degradation products of drugs using LC-MS tools: application to piroxicam and meloxycam, Anal. Methods 3 (2011) 2864–2872.

[34] S.G. Jivani, V.J. Stella, Mechanism of decarboxylation of p-aminosalicylic acid, J. Pharm. Sci. 74 (1985) 1274–1282.

[35] D.C. Monkhouse, L. Van Campen, A.J. Aguiar, Kinetics of dehydration and isomerization of prostaglandins E_1 and E_2, J. Pharm. Sci. 62 (1973) 576–580.

[36] G.F. Thomson, J.M. Collins, L.M. Schmalzried, Total rate equation for decompostion of prostaglandin E_2, J. Pharm. Sci. 62 (1973) 1738–1739.

[37] H. Bundgaard, Polymerization of penicillins: kinetics and mechanism of di- and polymerization of ampicillin in aqueous solution, Acta Pharm. Suec. 13 (1976) 9–26.

CHAPTER 4

Drug Degradation in Semisolid Dosage Forms

Drug degradation in semisolid dosage forms frequently resembles drug degradation in solutions, especially in those dosage forms that consist of one liquid phase, such as gels. *Gels* are semisolid drug dosage forms that can be as soft as jelly or as hard as solids. They mainly consist of liquid, but behave like solids due to a three-dimensional network within the liquid. Thus, from a drug stability point of view, gels are single-phase liquid states. For example, hydrogels can consist of 99.9% water and only 0.1% water-soluble polymers that form the network. Drug degradation in hydrogels follows the same kinetics and degradation mechanisms as in aqueous solutions. Organogels (sometimes referred to as oleogels or lipogels) are gels in which the homogeneous liquid phase consists of a nonaqueous solvent, such as an organic solvent, a mineral oil, or a vegetable oil. *Ointments* consist of single-phase bases in which drugs are dispersed. Ointment bases can consist of liquid paraffins or vegetable oils with emulsifying agents (water-emulsifying ointments) or without emulsifying agents (hydrophobic ointments), or with water-soluble bases, such as macrogols (hydrophilic ointments). Water-emulsifying and hydrophilic ointments may contain some water. *Creams* are emulsions consisting of a lipophilic phase and an aqueous phase. Hydrophilic creams are o/w emulsions (oil is the dispersed, and water the continuous, phase) and lipophilic creams are w/o emulsions (water is the dispersed, and oil is the continuous, phase). Ointments can contain drug suspensions in which case the drug is partly in a solid phase. The drug degradation kinetics will then be similar to those of aqueous drug suspensions (see Chapter 2, Section 2.1 Zero-order reactions). In creams, the drug is dispersed between the oil phase and the aqueous phase, and frequently the drug degrades much faster in the aqueous phase than in the oil phase. The observed rate constant for degradation is the weighted average of the rate constants of the oil and aqueous phases (see Chapter 2, Section 2.11 Disperse colloidal systems).

4.1 TRETINOIN

Tretinoin (all-trans-retinoic acid) is marketed as a hydrogel containing 0.05% w/v of dissolved tretinoin in a base consisting of aqueous ethanolic (15% w/w) solution embedded in a polyacrylate matrix. When the gel is exposed to light, tretinoin can be isomerized to form isotretinoin (13-cis-retinoic acid) [1]:

Tretinoin   Light →   Isotretinoin

4.2 BETAMETHASONE 17-VALERATE

Corticosteroid 17α-monoesters are unstable and readily rearrange to form the corresponding 21-monoesters. Thus, in aqueous solutions and semisolid dosage forms, betamethasone 17-valerate rearranges to form betamethasone 21-valerate:

Bethamethasone 17-ester   →   Bethamethasone 21-ester

Betamethasone 21-valerate is then hydrolyzed to form the alcohol. The pH-rate profile for the rate of disappearance of betamethasone 17-valerate in aqueous solutions is shown in Fig. 4.1. The profile shows that the drug has maximum stability at a pH between 3 and 4. Rearrangement from the 17-ester to the 21-ester is known to occur in both ointments and creams [3]. Dilution of betamethasone 17-valerate cream with a base having a neutral or alkaline pH can accelerate the drug degradation (Fig. 4.1).

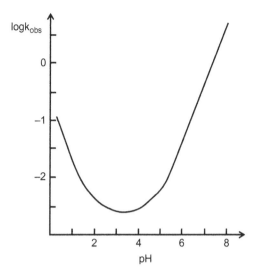

Figure 4.1 Sketch of the pH-rate profile for the degradation of betamethasone 17-valerate in aqueous solution at 60°C (I = 0.5). The observed rate constant has the units of h⁻¹ [2].

REFERENCES

[1] A. Bargagna, E. Martani, S. Dorato, TLC, HPTLC and HPLC determination of cis- and trans-retinoic acids, retinol and retinyl acetate in topically applied products, Acta Technol. Legis Medicam. 2 (1991) 75−85.

[2] H. Bundgaard, J. Hansen, Studies on the stability of corticosteroids. VI. Kinetics of the rearrangement of betamethasone-17-valerate to the 21-valerate ester in aqueous solution, Int. J. Pharm. 7 (1981) 197−203.

[3] Y.W. Yip, A.L.W. Po, The stability of betamethasone-17-valerate in semi-solid bases, J. Pharm. Pharmacol. 31 (1979) 400−402.

CHAPTER 5

Stability of Peptides and Proteins

Peptides and proteins are subjected to chemical degradation in much the same way as low molecular weight drugs. In addition, peptides and proteins can be subjected to physical degradation (i.e., alteration of their higher order structures (Fig. 5.1)). The primary protein structure refers to the amino acid sequence of the polypeptide chain. The amino acids are held together by relatively strong covalent bonds. The secondary structure refers to the regular substructures of compounds, such as the alpha helix and beta-sheet. The secondary structure is held together by hydrogen bonds that are relatively weak. The tertiary structure is the three-dimensional structure of a single protein molecule where, for example, hydrophobic moieties are buried within the protein structure and held together by relatively weak hydrophobic interactions. Enhanced stability can be obtained via salt bridges, hydrogen bonds, and covalent disulfide bonds. Quaternary protein structure is the three-dimensional structure of a multisubunit protein. The quaternary structure is held together by salt bridges, hydrogen bonds, and/or disulfide bonds.

5.1 PHYSICAL DEGRADATION

Physical degradation of peptides and proteins involves changes in their secondary, tertiary, or quaternary structures (i.e., the loss of their native three-dimensional structures). *Denaturation* can be due to increases in temperature, pH changes that alter the ionization of carboxylic acids and amino acids, changes in ionic strength, and changes from an aqueous to an organic solution media. Denaturation frequently leads to the loss of specific biological activity. *Aggregation* can be due to the rearrangement of hydrophobic protein moieties in such a manner that two or more protein molecules associate to form an aggregate that can possibly lead to precipitation. Interfacial protein adsorption may enhance aggregation and precipitation. Both denaturation and aggregation may be reversible, although they are most often irreversible. Enhanced physical stability can be obtained through the prevention or the reduction of protein adsorption to surfaces and the minimization of protein exposure

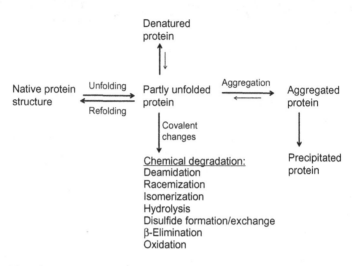

Figure 5.1 Scheme showing the main degradation pathways of proteins.

to air. Polyalcohols, such as sorbitol and glycerol, are known to bind to the protein surface and protect its three-dimensional structure. Other excipients may enhance protein stability by protecting its hydration or by some other mechanisms. It is also important to adjust the pH and salt content of aqueous protein and peptide solutions.

5.2 CHEMICAL DEGRADATION

The chemical degradation of peptides and proteins occurs through similar mechanisms to the degradation of small drug molecules, and they are affected by temperature and pH, as previously described in Chapter 2. However, their degradation is also affected by their amino acid composition, sequence, and conformation. For example, *deamidation* is the hydrolysis of a side chain amide in asparagine or glutamine residue to form a free carboxylic acid. Deamidation is a specific acid/base catalyzed reaction that displays a pH of optimum stability. Insulin is an example of a drug that undergoes deamidation in aqueous solutions [1]. All amino acid residues except glycine possess a chiral carbon atom and are subject to specific acid/base catalyzed *racemization* and *isomerization*. Peptides and proteins in all living organisms consist exclusively of the L-forms of amino acids (except in certain types of bacteria). However, after death, proteins and peptides are slowly racemized and by determining the D/L amino acid ratio of archeological specimens, it is possible to estimate how long ago the specimen died [2].

The same applies to natural peptides and protein used in medicine. They are mainly of the L configuration, but are relatively rapidly isomerized under alkaline conditions. *Hydrolysis* is commonly observed during peptide and protein degradation. Nonenzymatic hydrolysis of the peptide bonds within a protein's primary structure (i.e., fragmentation of the proteins) releases polypeptides. Aspartic acid bonds, such as the Asp−Gly and Asp−Pro peptide bonds, are the type most susceptible to hydrolytic cleavage, primarily at the C-terminus and then at the N-terminus [3]. *Proteolysis* is hydrolysis (or cleavage by other means) of proteins into smaller polypeptides and/or amino acids.

Disulfide bonds play an important role in the three-dimensional structure and stability of some proteins [4]. Thus, formation of the disulfide bonds or changes in the disulfide bonds (e.g., disulfide bond scrambling) can lead to changes in the secondary or tertiary structure and loss of biological activity. For example, human insulin requires the correct formation of both intra- and interchain disulfide bonds to function properly [5]. Disulfide-linked insulin dimers are, for example, known to be formed in parenteral formulations. *β-Elimination* can occur in amino acids that have β side chains such as Cys, Ser, Thr, Phe, and Lys, and the reaction is influenced by pH, temperature, and the presence of metal ions. This can have a significant effect on the stability and biological activity of proteins such as immunoglobulins [6]. Inactivation of proteins at elevated temperatures can be due to β-elimination of disulfide bonds from a cysteine residue. *Oxidation* is one of the major degradation pathways of peptides and proteins and occurs when oxygen radicals react with certain amino acids such as the sulfur atoms of Met and Cys and the aromatic rings of His, Trp, and Tyr.

5.3 INSULIN

The human insulin molecule (MW 5808 g/mol) consists of 52 amino acid residues in two polypeptide chains, chain A (21 residues) and B (31 residues), that are linked by two disulfide bonds in addition to one disulfide loop in chain A. Insulin is characterized as a small globular protein. It is slightly soluble in water but practically insoluble in organic solvents like ethanol. The stability of insulin has been evaluated both in aqueous solutions and in the solid state [7–9]. Insulin from sources other than humans (e.g., bovine and porcine insulins) have a slightly different primary structure, but all have basically the same secondary and tertiary structure. The quaternary structure is formed through self-association of insulin monomers. Insulin monomers only exist in very dilute solutions. In more concentrated solutions (like most pharmaceutical preparations), dimers are formed and, under certain conditions and especially if zinc ions are present, three dimers self-associate to form a hexamer. Crystalline insulin hexamers are the most common solid form found in pharmaceutical products.

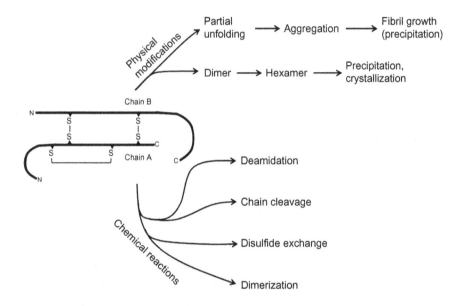

Physical modifications: Globular proteins, like insulin, tend to form somewhat hydrophilic spherical structures with lipophilic moieties buried within the structure. When an aqueous insulin solution comes into contact with hydrophobic surfaces (i.e., air–water or plastic–water interphases), the three-dimensional insulin structure tends to unfold, resulting in hydrophobic interactions (i.e., aggregation) of the partial unfolded insulin chains with consequent precipitation of insulin fibrils. The addition of small amounts of lecithins and/or metal ions such as Ca^{++} and Zn^{++} can prevent the formation of insulin fibrils in aqueous insulin solutions.

Chemical reactions: The two main chemical degradation mechanisms are hydrolysis (i.e., deamidation and chain cleavage) and intermolecular reactions (i.e., formation of covalently linked insulin dimers and polymers). For aqueous insulin solutions or suspensions, under neutral or weakly basic conditions, the deamidation proceeds through a cyclic imide intermediate:

Hydrolytic cleavage of the A chain is observed in aqueous rhombohedral crystalline insulin suspensions in the presence of free zinc ions. The intermolecular reactions proceed in general at much slower rates than the hydrolytic reactions. In addition to covalent insulin dimers, oligomers, and polymers, insulin is known to form covalent insulin–protamine products in pharmaceutical preparations that contain protamine. The maximum insulin stability against hydrolysis and the formation of oligomers and polymers appears to be at a pH between 6 and 7.

The main degradation pathway of insulin in parenteral formulations is hydrolysis. The deamidation products have essentially the same potency as the intact insulin molecule. The extent of deamidation during the shelf-life of the product (2 years at $2-8°C$) is $\leq 7\%$, resulting in insignificant changes in potency. Hydrolysis of the peptide chain results in products that possess only about 2% of the insulin potency. However, when stored at $2-8°C$, the decrease in potency is less than 5% during the product's shelf-life [7].

Question 5.1: What is the difference between an intermolecular reaction and an intramolecular reaction? What is the difference between intermolecular catalysis and intramolecular catalysis?

REFERENCES

[1] R.T. Darrington, B.D. Anderson, Evidence for a common intermediate in insulin deamidation and covalent dimer formation: effects of pH and aniline trapping in dilute acidic solutions, J. Pharm. Sci. 84 (1995) 275–282.

[2] J.L. Bada, Amino acid racemization dating of fossil bones, Ann. Rev. Earth Planet. Sci. 13 (1985) 241–268.

[3] M. Seo, J. Kim, S. Park, J.H. Lee, T. Kim, J. Lee, J. Kim, Weak acid hydrolysis of proteins, Bull. Korean Chem. Soc. 34 (2013) 27–28.

[4] L. Zhang, C.P. Chou, M. Moo-Young, Disulfide bond formation and its impact on the biological activity and stability of recombinant therapeutic proteins produced by Escherichia coli expression system, Biotechnol. Adv. 29 (2011) 923–929.

[5] Z.S. Qiao, C.Y. Min, Q.X. Hua, M.A. Weiss, Y.M. Feng, In vitro refolding of human proinsulin—kinetic intermediates, putative disulfide-forming pathway, folding initiation site, and potential role of C-peptide in folding process, J. Biol. Chem. 278 (2003) 17800–17809.

[6] H.-C. Liu, K. May, Disulfide bond structures of IgG molecules. Structural variations, chemical modifications and possible impacts to stability and biological function, MABS 4 (2012) 17–23.

[7] J. Brange, L. Langkjær, Insulin structure and stability, Pharm. Biotechnol. 5 (1993) 315–350.

[8] R.G. Strickley, B.D. Anderson, Solid-state stability of human insulin I. Mechanism and the effect of water on the kinetics of degradation in lyophiles from pH 2–5 solutions, Pharm. Res. 13 (1996) 1142–1153.

[9] R.G. Strickley, B.D. Anderson, Solid-state stability of human insulin II. Effect of water on reactive intermediate partitioning in lyophiles from pH 2–5 solutions: stabilization against covalent dimer formation, J. Pharm. Sci. 86 (1997) 645–653.

CHAPTER 6

Drug Degradation in Solid State

Most drugs are in the solid form at room temperature, and most drugs are administered in their solid dosage forms. The most common pharmaceutical dosage form by far is the tablet. Thus, the evaluation of solid-state stability is a very important aspect of drug stability.

Solid-state drug degradation can be divided into physical degradation and chemical degradation. No covalent bonds are formed or broken during physical degradation of drug substances. Frequently, physical degradation involves polymorphic transformations in which unstable crystal structures or amorphic forms are transformed into more stable crystal structures. Physical degradation sometimes involves desolvation reactions in which crystal solvents, such as water, are removed from the solid drug (e.g., pseudopolymorphic transformations). The more stable crystal structures (having higher melting points) have, in general, lower aqueous solubilities than corresponding unstable structures (having lower melting points). Thus, these physical transformations can lead to decreased drug bioavailability, since only dissolved drug molecules are able to permeate biological membranes. Chemical degradation involves breakage and/or formation of covalent bonds (e.g., hydrolysis, oxidation, photochemical decomposition, and pyrolysis). It mainly occurs in a solution phase and most often follows pseudo-zero-order kinetics. Moisture present in the solid dosage form (e.g., crystal water, residual moisture from manufacturing, or absorbed atmospheric moisture) or from the melting of excipients or melting of the drug itself, can serve as a microscopic solution phase in which the drug degradation mainly occurs within the solid dosage form [1–4]. Previously, degradation of aspirin in solid dosage forms has been described (see Section 3.1.1 and Fig. 3.6). The following are a few additional examples.

6.1 CHLORAMPHENICOL PALMITATE

Chloramphenicol palmitate is known to exist in four different solid states: an amorphous form and three crystal forms, polymorphs A, B, and C.

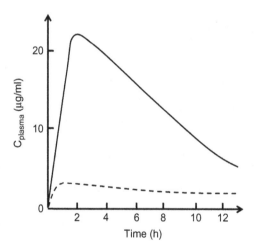

Polymorph A is the most thermodynamically stable form. It has the highest melting point and the slowest dissolution rate. Polymorph B has a somewhat lower melting point and is dissolved much faster. Polymorph C is the most unstable form and is relatively rapidly converted to polymorph B, for example, during grinding [5]. Polymorph B is then converted to the most stable form polymorph A. The commercial form of chloramphenicol palmitate is polymorph B, which has relatively good bioavailability after oral administration, while polymorph A has much lower bioavailability (Fig. 6.1).

Figure 6.1 Sketch of plasma concentration profile of chloramphenicol after administration of chloramphenicol palmitate, equivalent to 1.5 grams of chloramphenicol, in an aqueous oral suspension to humans. Polymorph A (broken curve); polymorph B (solid curve) [6].

6.2 NITROGLYCERIN

Nitroglycerin (melting point 14°C) is a liquid at room temperature. Nitroglycerin is lipophilic and a volatile compound. It is an ester that undergoes specific base catalyzed hydrolysis in aqueous solutions, but is relatively stable under acidic conditions. However, the drug is poorly soluble in water (solubility is about 1 mg/ml). Decreased potency of

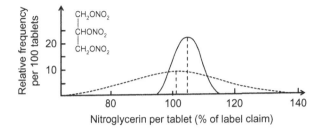

Figure 6.2 Content uniformity for conventional sublingual nitroglycerin tablets at the time of manufacturing (solid curve) and after storage for 5 months at 25°C (broken curve) [7].

nitroglycerin sublingual tablets is mainly due to evaporation of nitroglycerin from the tablets (Fig. 6.2).

In conventional tablets (i.e., tablets without stabilizers), nitroglycerin evaporates from one tablet and enters into another, leading to uneven drug distribution from one tablet to another (Fig. 6.2). Furthermore, nitroglycerin migrates relatively easily from tablets to various materials such as paper, plastic, and cotton. The addition of excipients (i.e. stabilizers) to the tablets that lower the vapor pressure of nitroglycerin, such as the addition of 0.5 to 2% polyvinylpyrrolidone (polyvidone), has been shown to decrease nitroglycerin evaporation and migration [8]. Nitroglycerin sublingual tablets that are currently on the market contain stabilizers that enhance their physical stability.

6.3 CHEMICAL DEGRADATION

Chemical drug degradation in solid dosage forms, such as tablets, most frequently occurs in microscopic drug solutions within the dosage form, and most frequently these microscopic drug solutions are aqueous solutions. One example of this type of solid-state hydrolysis is the solid-state hydrolysis of aspirin (see Section 3.1.1). Another example is the solid-state hydrolysis of meclofenoxate hydrochloride (Fig. 6.3).

As in the case of aspirin (Fig. 3.6), meclofenoxate hydrolysis occurs in the microscopic water domains (or microscopic pools) within the solid dosage form or the pure solid drug powder. The size of these water domains will increase with increasing relative humidity (RH) and, thus, the rate of degradation in the solid state will increase with increasing RH. Furthermore, both aqueous drug solubility and the value of the rate constant will increase with

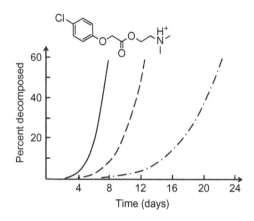

Figure 6.3 Sketch of the solid state hydrolysis of meclofenoxate hydrochloride at different relative humidity (RH) and temperature: 60°C, 49.9% RH (solid curve); 60°C, 43.1% RH (broken curve); 50°C, 49.7% RH (double broken curve) [9]. The lag time was estimated to be 5, 9 and 15 h respectively.

increasing temperature. When a dry solid drug sample is placed in a chamber of fixed temperature and RH, the sample will absorb water from the atmosphere within the chamber until equilibrium has been reached. The solid drug will dissolve in the water domain until saturation concentration has been reached ($[A]_{sat}$ in Eq. 3.8). Then the solid-state degradation will proceed at a constant rate (k_{solid} in Eq. 3.8). The time it takes to reach this steady-state degradation represents the lag time (i.e., the extension of the linear degradation profile to the x-axis in Fig. 6.3).

Solid-state degradation of cephalosporins has been shown to depend on the type of crystal structure, the amorphic form displaying the fastest degradation, as well as the moisture content and temperature [10]. The rate of solid-state oxidation of ascorbic acid also depends on the moisture content and temperature, as well as on the presence of atmospheric oxygen [11]. In general, when degradation occurs in microscopic water domains (i.e., microscopic aqueous pools) within the solid material, the degradation rate depends on 1) the moisture content of the solid material, 2) the solubility of a given drug in the water domains, and 3) the temperature. The moisture content is affected by the presence of hygroscopic excipients and the RH. The solubility, especially of ionizable drugs, in the water domains can be affected by excipients. Temperature will affect both the drug solubility and the value of the reaction-rate constant, both of which increase with increasing temperature. Chemical degradation in the solid state can also proceed in nonaqueous liquid domains as well as in true solid states.

Question 6.1: Guillory and Higuchi studied the solid-state degradation of various vitamin A derivatives in open containers at 50°C and drew the following plot showing the relationship between the logarithm of the zero-order vitamin A degradation constant (logk where k is in mol/h) and the melting point (T in Kelvin) of the derivatives [1]. Explain the relationship.

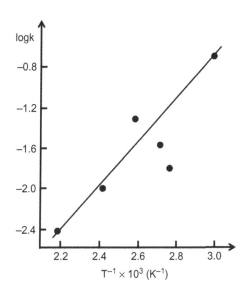

REFERENCES

[1] J.K. Guillory, T. Higuchi, Solid state stability of some crystalline vitamin A compounds, J. Pharm. Sci. 51 (1962) 100–105.

[2] J.T. Carstensen, Stability of solids and solid dosage forms, J. Pharm. Sci. 63 (1974) 1–14.

[3] B.D. Glass, C. Novák, E.M. Brown, The thermal and photostability of solid pharmaceuticals – A review, J. Therm. Anal. Cal. 77 (2004) 1013–1036.

[4] A.S. Narang, D. Desai, S. Badawy, Impact of excipient interactions on solid dosage form stability, Pharm. Res. 29 (2012) 2660–2683.

[5] M. Otsuka, N. Kaneniwa, Effect of seed crystals on solid-state transformation of polymorphs of chloramphenicol palmitate during grinding, J. Pharm. Sci. 75 (1986) 506–511.

[6] A.J. Aguiar, J. Krc, A.W. Kinkel, J.C. Samyn, Effect of polymorphism on the absorption of chloramphenicol from chloramphenicol palmitate, J. Pharm. Sci. 56 (1967) 847–853.

[7] S.A. Fusari, Nitroglycerin sublingual tablets I: stability of conventional tablets, J. Pharm. Sci. 62 (1973) 122–129.

[8] M.J. Pikal, D.A. Bibler, B. Rutherford, Polymer sorption of nitroglycerin and stability of molden nitroglycerin tablets in unit-dose packaging, J. Pharm. Sci. 66 (1977) 1293–1297.

[9] S. Yoshioka, M. Uchiyama, Nonlinear estimation of kinetic parameters for solid-state hydrolysis of water-soluble drugs, J. Pharm. Sci. 75 (1986) 459–462.

[10] M.J. Pikal, K.M. Dellerman, Stability testing of pharmaceuticals by high-sensitivity isothermal calorimetry at 25°C: cephalosporins in the solid and aqueous solution ststes, Int. J. Pharm. 50 (1989) 233–252.

[11] R.J. Willson, A.E. Beezer, J.C. Mitchell, Solid state reactions studied by isothermal microcalorimetry; the solid state oxidation of ascorbic acid, Int. J. Pharm. 132 (1996) 45–51.

CHAPTER 7

Stability Testing

Stability testing of drugs and drug products is required to ensure the integrity of pharmaceutical products. Testing is carried out mainly during product development and registration, but also after the products have been marketed. A drug product should retain its physical (e.g., appearance, dissolution, and uniformity), chemical (e.g., potency), microbial (e.g., sterility or resistance to microbial growth), therapeutic (i.e., therapeutic efficacy), and toxicological (i.e., no increase in toxicity) quality during its shelf-life. During product development, accelerated stability tests are performed as a part of stability optimization (e.g., selection of excipients, pH, medium, and package), and also to determine storage conditions and to obtain a provisional shelf-life for the product. *Accelerated testing* is, in general, performed at elevated temperatures and the Arrhenius equation is used to predict the shelf-life at room temperature or with respect to other potential storage conditions, such as refrigeration. The shelf-life of the finished pharmaceutical product is then determined under proposed storage conditions with final packaging. It is based on *long-term (real-time) stability studies* on a number of batches. Regulatory agencies, such as the European Medicines Agency (EMA) and the Federal Drug Administration (FDA), require data from such studies to be included in registration applications. A specific, stability-indicating assay for quantitative determination of the drug substance (i.e., the active pharmaceutical ingredient, or API) must be included in registration applications for all new drug products. Frequently, it is possible to employ the same analytical procedure (e.g., high performance liquid chromatography, or HPLC) for both the assay of the drug substance and the quantitation of impurities.

7.1 GUIDELINES FOR STABILITY TESTING

Stability testing of new active pharmaceutical ingredients and finished pharmaceutical products has been harmonized at a global level. The World Health Organization (WHO) has published guidelines that are available at WHO's website (www.who.int). The main guidelines are, however, found at the ICH (the International Conference on the

Harmonisation of Technical Requirements for Registration of Pharmaceuticals for Human Use) homepage (www.ich.org). ICH brings together the drug regulatory authorities of Europe (www.ema. europa.eu), Japan (www.pmda.go.jp), and the United States (www.fda. gov). In addition, the Association of South East Asian Nations (www. asean.org) has harmonized stability testing of pharmaceutical products. Although most regional areas of the world follow the ICH stability guidelines, they do sometimes deviate from the ICH guidelines and may post some additional requirements. The WHO guidelines do also in some cases differ from the ICH guidelines [1]. The ICH stability guidelines consist of numerous publications, including:

- Q1A(R2) Stability Testing of New Drug Substances and Products,
- Q1B Stability Testing: Photostability Testing of New Drug Substances and Products,
- Q1C Stability Testing for New Dosage Forms,
- Q1D Bracketing and Matrixing Designs for Stability Testing of New Drug Substances and Products,
- Q1E Evaluation of Stability Data,
- Q1F Stability Data Package for Registration Applications in Climatic Zones III and IV, and
- Q5C Stability testing of Biotechnological/Biological Products.

A brief summary of the ICH guidelines is given in Table 7.1. According to the ICH, the purpose of stability testing of pure drugs and pharmaceutical products is to provide evidence of how the quality of drug substances and drug products change with time under the influence of a variety of environmental factors such as temperature, humidity, and light. Stress testing of drug substances, excipients, and drug products are used to identify degradation pathways and degradation products (potential impurities), as well as the intrinsic stability of the compounds under various conditions. For example, stress tests of a drug substance (i.e., an active pharmaceutical ingredient (API)) are performed at temperatures above those used during accelerated stability testing, for example at $\geq 50°C$ in $10°C$ increments (e.g., 50, 60, and $70°C$) and at $\geq 75\%$ relative humidity (RH). When appropriate, oxidation and photolysis studies should also be performed. Stress testing may include the following:

1. Degradation studies in an aqueous hydrochloric acid solution,
2. Degradation studies in an aqueous sodium hydroxide solution,
3. Degradation studies in the presence of hydrogen peroxide,

Table 7.1 Brief Summary of the ICH Guidelines for Testing of Drug Substances and New Drug Products.

Parameter	ICH Stability Testing Requirements	
	Drug Substances[1]	Drug Products[2]
Batch selection:	Data from three primary batches are required	
Container closure system:	The stability studies should be conducted on the drug substance packed in the same container closure system as proposed for storage and distribution	The stability studies should be conducted on the drug product packed in the same container closure system, i.e. both primary and secondary, as proposed for marketing
Specifications:	Combination of physical, chemical, biological and microbiological tests and acceptances criteria that the drug substance/product should meet throughout its shelf-life	
Testing frequency:	Accelerated: 0, 3 and 6 months Intermediate: 0, 6, 9 and 12 months Long term: 0, 3, 6, 9, 12, 18 and 24 months and then every 12 months through the proposed re-testing period	
General storage conditions:	Accelerated: $40 \pm 2°C/75 \pm 5\%$ RH Intermediate: $30 \pm 2°C/65 \pm 5\%$ RH Long term: $25 \pm 2°C/60 \pm 5\%$ RH or $30 \pm 2°C/65 \pm 5\%$ RH	
Refrigerator storage conditions:	Accelerated: $25 \pm 2°C/60 \pm 5\%$ RH Long term: $5 \pm 3°C$	
Freezer storage conditions:	Long term: $-20 \pm 5°C$	
Stability commitment:	If the long term data on does not cover the proposed substance re-test period or product shelf-life granted at the time of approval then a commitment should be made to continue the stability studies to firmly establish the re-test period or shelf-life.	
Evaluation:	Based on the evaluation of the stability data the re-test period of a drug substance or the shelf-life of a drug product should be established.	
Photostability:	For drug substances, photostability testing should consist of two parts: forced degradation testing and confirmatory testing relating to normal handling of the substance.	i) Test on the exposed drug product, then if necessary ii) test on the product in primary package, and then if necessary iii) test on the product in the marketing package.
	The light source can be an artificial daylight fluorescent lamp combining visible and ultraviolet outputs.	

[1]ICH: the unformulated drug substance that may subsequently be formulated with excipients to produce the dosage form.
[2]ICH: The dosage form (e.g. tablet, capsule, solution, cream, eye drops) in the final immediate packaging intended for marketing.

4. Photostability studies (e.g., in sunlight or under a UV light), and
5. Evaluation of stability during sterilization (e.g., during heating in an autoclave).

Stability testing of the finished pharmaceutical product should be conducted on the product as packaged in the container closure system proposed for marketing, including both the primary and secondary packaging with labels. The storage conditions displayed on the labeling should be based on these stability studies of the drug product.

It should be mentioned that although normal manufacturing and analytical variations are to be expected, it is important that a drug product provides 100 percent of the labeled amount of the drug substance at the time of batch release.

7.2 DORZOLAMIDE EYE DROPS

Dorzolamide ((4S,6S)-4-(ethylamino)-6-methyl-5,6-dihydro-4H-thieno [2,3-b]thiopyran-2-sulfonamide 7,7-dioxide) has two pKa values (i.e., 6.4 and 8.5). It is mainly in its cationic form at a pH below 6.4, mainly unionized at a pH between 6.4 and 8.5, and mainly in its anionic form at a pH above 8.5. At room temperature, its aqueous solubility is about 40 mg/ml at pH <5.5 and about 4 mg/ml at pH 7.4 [2,3]. Dorzolamide has maximum stability at a pH between 4 and 6 [4]. Due to photochemical instability, aqueous dorzolamide eyedrops should be stored in light-resistant containers at 15–30°C. The commercial product is an isotonic aqueous solution containing 20 mg/ml dorzolamide at pH 5.6. Stress tests have shown, according to the European Pharmacopoeia, that the main impurities found in aqueous dorzolamide solutions (Fig. 7.1) are impurity A ((4R,6R)-4-(ethylamino)-6-methyl-5,6-dihydro-4H-thieno[2,3-b]thiopyran-2-sulfonamide 7,7-dioxide), impurity B consisting of enantiomers ((4RS,6SR)-4-(ethylamino)-6-methyl-5,6-dihydro-4H-thieno[2,3-b]thiopyran-2-sulfonamide 7,7-dioxide), impurity C ([2-[[(4S,6S)-6-methyl-7,7-dioxo-2-sulfamoyl-4,5,6,7-tetra-hydro-7λ^6-thieno[2,3-b]thiopyran-4-yl]amino]ethyl]boronic acid), and impurity D ((4S,6S)-4-amino-6-methyl-5,6-dihydro-4H-thieno[2,3-b] thiopyran-2-sulfonamide 7,7-dioxide). The analytical method used for the quantitative determination of dorzolamide has to be able to separate the impurities from the active compound. It is not sufficient to determine the characteristics for only the active compound; the identity and the amount of the different impurities also have to be determined. According to the European Pharmacopoeia, the maximum allowable amount of impurity A in the drug substance (dorzolamide) is 0.5%. The maximum allowable amount of the other impurities is 0.3%, including a maximum of 0.15% of impurity C. The maximum amount of impurity A in an aqueous dorzolamide eyedrop solution is frequently set at 1.0%, and the

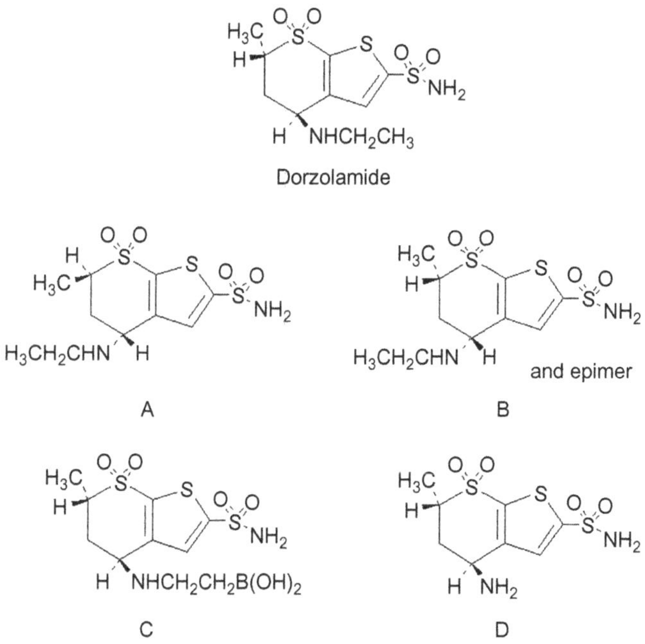

Figure 7.1 The chemical structure of dorzolamide and the four impurities (A, B, C and D) identified by the European Pharmacopoeia.

total amount of other related substances is set at 4.0%, including a maximum of 1% of impurity of C. The dorzolamide content of the eyedrops should be between 95 and 105% of the labeled amount.

In addition, aqueous dorzolamide eyedrop solutions have to pass other tests and requirements, such as those for pH, viscosity, osmolality, particle size, and sterility.

REFERENCES

[1] H. Patel, B.R. Sudeendra, V. Balamuralidhara, K.T.M. Pramod, Comparison of stability testing requirements of ICH with other international regulatory agencies, Pharma Times 43(9) (2011) 21–34.

[2] H.H. Sigurdsson, E. Stefánsson, E. Gudmundsdóttir, T. Eysteinsson, M. Thorsteinsdóttir, T. Loftsson, Cyclodextrin formulation of dorzolamide and its distribution in the eye after topical administration, J. Control. Rel. 102 (2005) 255–262.

[3] T. Loftsson, P. Jansook, E. Stefánsson, Topical drug delivery to the eye: dorzolamide, Acta Ophthalmol. 90 (2012) 603–608.

[4] C.-H. Chiang, C.-H. Hsieh, D.-W. Lu, K.-D. Kao, Stability of topical carbonic anhydrase inhibitor 6-hydroxyethoxy-2-benzothiazole sulfonamide, J. Pharm. Sci. 81 (1992) 299–302.

CHAPTER 8

Problems

The following problems are based on experimental data extracted from various original research publications in international peer-reviewed journals. In many cases the data shown has been modified from the original data and, thus, does not show the normal experimental variation frequently observed in such data.

8.1 RACEMIZATION OF (R)-OXAZEPAM

Aso et al. [1] studied the racemization of (R)-oxazepam in an aqueous solution at pH 12 and 0°C. Their results are displayed in the table below. Calculate t_{90}.

Time (min)	% (R)-Oxazepam
15	86.6
30	76.8
45	69.6
60	64.4

8.2 CONSECUTIVE DEGRADATION OF PROSTAGLANDIN

Prostaglandin degrades in an aqueous solution at pH 8.0 and 60°C as follows:

The table below shows how the PGA_2 concentration changes with time. The initial PGE_2 ($=[A]_0$) was 0.100 M and the initial PGA_2 was 0.000 M. Calculate k_1 and k_2. What is the shelf-life (t_{90}) of PGE_2 at these conditions?

Time (h)	$[PGA_2] \times 10^2$ (M)
1	1.71
2	3.10
5	5.82
10	7.55
20	7.41
40	5.28
60	3.65
80	2.52
100	1.74

8.3 EFFECT OF BUFFER SALTS ON LOMUSTINE DEGRADATION

Various pharmaceutical excipients, such as buffer salts and water-soluble polymers, can affect drug degradation through the formation of drug/excipient complexes. When the anticancer drug lomustine was dissolved in an aqueous solution containing Tris buffer (pH 8.0 and 55°C), it was observed that Tris decreased the degradation rate through the formation of a lomustine/Tris (1:1) complex [2]. Calculate k_c and $K_{1:1}$ for the complex.

[Tris] (M)	k_{obs} (min^{-1})
0.000	0.4234
0.050	0.2856
0.125	0.2482
0.175	0.2251
0.250	0.2137
0.500	0.2044

8.4 pH-RATE PROFILE FOR AMOXICILLIN

Zia et al. [3] determined the pH-rate profile for amoxicillin at zero buffer concentration and 35°C (I = 0.5), and the following degradation rate constants were calculated based on their results:

(See also section 3.1.4 β-Lactam antibiotics)

At 35°C and I = 0.5:

$pKa_1 = 2.87$
$pKa_2 = 7.28$
$pKa_3 = 9.65$
$pK_w = [H^+] \times [OH^-] = 13.6$

pH	k_{obs} (h^{-1})
1.00	15.31×10^{-2}
1.50	6.166×10^{-2}
2.00	3.236×10^{-2}
2.50	1.905×10^{-2}
3.00	1.023×10^{-2}
3.50	0.447×10^{-2}
4.00	0.158×10^{-2}
5.00	0.170×10^{-2}
6.00	0.158×10^{-2}
7.00	1.445×10^{-2}
7.50	2.140×10^{-2}
8.00	3.236×10^{-2}
9.00	5.012×10^{-2}
10.00	32.36×10^{-2}

A. Draw the pH-rate profile for amoxicillin at 35°C.
B. Determine the rate equation for amoxicillin from the pH-rate profile, and calculate the rate constants for specific acid, specific base, and uncatalyzed degradation.
C. k_{obs} is $1.70 \times 10^{-3} h^{-1}$ at pH 5.0 and 35°C. The Ea value of the rate constant is 18.1 kcal/mol. Estimate $\Delta G^{\neq}$, the probability factor (P), and $\Delta S^{\neq}$.

8.5 EFFECT OF GLUCOSE ON AMOXICILLIN DEGRADATION

It is common practice to dissolve antibiotics, such as β-lactams, into intravenous solutions. Isotonic glucose (dextrose) injections contain 5.0% (w/v) glucose. Glucose catalysis degradation of amoxicillin (see 3.1.4 β-Lactam antibiotics). The table shows the effect of glucose on the rate constant of amoxicillin degradation at pH 7.5 and 75°C. Write the rate equation and calculate the kinetic constants shown in the rate equation.

Glucose (% w/v)	Glucose (mol/liter)	k_{obs} (min^{-1})
0	0.000	$2.38\ 10^{-2}$
5	0.278	$8.18\ 10^{-2}$
10	0.556	$13.30\ 10^{-2}$

8.6 pH-RATE PROFILE AND SPECIFIC ACID/BASE CATALYSIS

The pH-rate profile of lithospermic acid B was determined in aqueous buffer solutions at 90°C and I = 0.50 (the unit of k_{obs} is h^{-1}), see table [4]. Determine the rate equation for amoxicillin from the pH-rate profile, and estimate the rate constants for specific acid, specific base, and uncatalyzed degradation. At 90°C, the pKa values of the acid are 3.14 and 5.52, and the value of pK_w is 12.45.

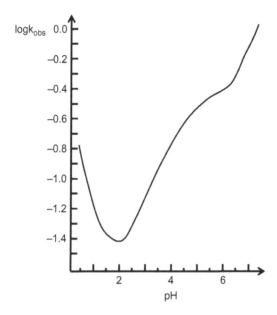

8.7 AZTREONAM POLYMERIZATION

Aztreonam is a monobactams antibiotic (see section 3.1.4 β-Lactam antibiotics) that forms dimers, trimers, and other oligomers in aqueous solutions. The sketch below shows the effect of initial aztreonam concentration on the formation of a polymeric product P in aqueous solution at pH 5.0 and 25°C [5]. Write the rate equation for the dimer and trimer formation. Why does the formation of P increase with an increase in the initial aztreonam concentration? Will the degradation rate be independent of the initial aztreonam concentration?

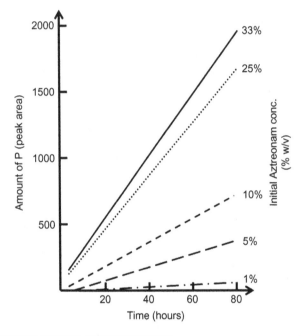

8.8 AQUEOUS DRUG SUSPENSION

An aqueous antibiotic suspension is to be prepared for oral delivery. The first-order degradation rate constant (k_{obs}) of the dissolved antibiotic in the media was determined to be 2.0×10^{-6} s^{-1} at pH 7.0 and 35°C. The solubility (S_0) of the antibiotic in the media was determined to be 10 mg/ml at pH 7.0 and 25°C. The total antibiotic concentration in the aqueous pH 7.0 suspension will be 25 mg/ml.

Estimate the shelf-life (t_{90}) of the aqueous antibiotic suspension at 25°C.

Estimate t_{90} at 5°C (i.e., refrigerator temperature), assuming that the antibiotic solubility will not change when the temperature is lowered.

8.9 RACEMIZATION OF ROPIVACAINE

Ropivacaine ((S)-N-(2,6-dimethylphenyl)-1-propylpiperidine-2-carbox-amide) undergoes racemization in aqueous solutions [6]. The results in the following table were obtained at 100°C and pH 5.5:

Time (Days)	% Ropivacaine (i.e., the S-form)
0.0	100.0
1.0	94.6
2.5	84.3
5.0	75.9
10	62.2
15	56.2

Calculate k_1 and k_{-1}. What is the shelf-life (t_{90}) at pH 5.5 and 100°C?

8.10 DEGRADATION OF SCOPOLAMINE

See the following table for the observed rate constants (k_{obs}) for the degradation of scopolamine at zero buffer concentration and 25°C [7, 8]. Scopolamine is only hydrolyzed at a pH below 3, but undergoes concurrent isomerization at a pH above 3. The hydrolysis accounts for 96% of the degradation at a pH between 3 and 7, but 72% at a pH above 8. Draw the pH-rate profile for scopolamine, determine the rate equation, and estimate the rate constants for specific acid, specific base, and uncatalyzed degradation. At 25°C, the pKa value of the hydrobromide is about 7.6, and the value of pK_w is 14.00.

pH	k_{obs} (h^{-1})
1.0	4.53×10^{-5}
2.0	3.60×10^{-6}
3.0	2.27×10^{-7}
3.7	5.71×10^{-8}
4.0	1.14×10^{-7}
5.0	1.14×10^{-6}
6.0	7.18×10^{-6}
7.0	7.18×10^{-5}
8.0	3.60×10^{-4}
9.0	1.80×10^{-3}
10.0	1.80×10^{-2}
11.0	1.80×10^{-1}

8.11 PRIMARY SALT EFFECT

The chemical stability of apaziquone (EO9) was investigated, including the influence of ionic strength at pH 4.0 and 25°C [9]:

I (mol/liter)	k_{obs} (s^{-1})
0.10	3.16×10^{-3}
0.25	7.94×10^{-3}
0.31	8.51×10^{-3}

Estimate the shelf-life of a dilute apaziquone pH 4.0 solution in pure water as well as in an aqueous 0.9% (w/v) NaCl solution.

8.12 LEAVING GROUPS

The sketch below shows the pH-rate profiles of aspirin (the solid line) and methylsalicylate (the broken line) at 25°C, where k_{obs} is min^{-1}. Determine the rate equations for aspirin and methylsalicylate. Why is methylsalicylate much less susceptible to hydrolysis at a pH below 8?

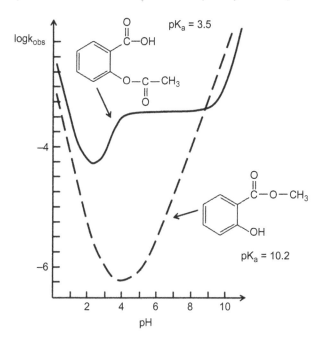

8.13 THE SHELF-LIFE OF TETRACYCLINE UNDER ACIDIC CONDITIONS

In an aqueous solution, tetracycline (TC), see section 3.3.4 and Fig. 3.17, undergoes both epimerization to form 4-epi-tetracycline (ETC) and dehydration to form anhydro-tetracycline (ATC) and then epi-anhydro-tetracycline (EATC):

$$
\begin{array}{ccc}
 & k_1 & \\
\text{TC} & \rightleftharpoons & \text{ETC} \\
 & k_{-1} & \\
\downarrow k_3 & & \downarrow k_4 \\
 & k_2 & \\
\text{ATC} & \rightleftharpoons & \text{EATC} \\
 & k_{-2} &
\end{array}
$$

The following rate constants were obtained at pH 1.5 and 60°C [10]:

$k_1 = 0.414\ \text{h}^{-1}$
$k_{-1} = 0.373\ \text{h}^{-1}$
$k_2 = 0.659\ \text{h}^{-1}$
$k_{-2} = 0.665\ \text{h}^{-1}$
$k_3 = 0.323\ \text{h}^{-1}$
$k_4 = 0.206\ \text{h}^{-1}$

Calculate the shelf-life (t_{90}) of tetracycline at pH 1.5 and 60°C.

8.14 PARENTERAL FORMULATION CONTAINING β-LACTAM ANTIBIOTIC

The following figure shows the pH-rate profile (k_{obs} in h^{-1}) and pH-solubility profile of a β-lactam antibiotic at 25°C. You are asked to formulate this drug as an aqueous parenteral solution containing 200 mg/ml of the drug without the usage of solubilizers such as surfactants, complexing agents, and organic solvents.

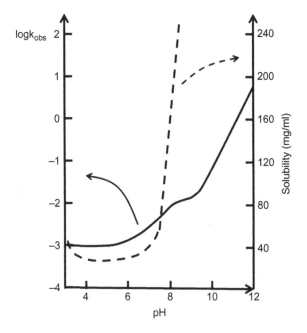

REFERENCES

[1] Y. Aso, S. Yoshioka, T. Shibazaki, M. Uchiyama, The kinetic of the rezemation of oxazepam in aqueous solution, Chem. Pharm. Bull. 36 (1988) 1834–1840.

[2] T. Loftsson, H. Fridriksdottir, Stabilizing effect of tris(hydroxymethyl)aminomethane (TRIS) on N-nitrosoureas in aqueous solutions, J. Pharm. Sci. 81 (1992) 197−198.

[3] H. Zia, N. Shalchian, F. Borhanian, Kinetics of amoxycillin degradation in aqueous solutions, Can. J. Pharm. Sci. 12 (1977) 80−83.

[4] Y.-X. Guo, Z.-L. Xiu, D.-J. Zhang, H. Wang, L.-X. Wang, H.-B. Xiao, Kinetics and mechanism of degradation of lithospermic acid B in aqueous solution, J. Pharm. Biom. Anal. 43 (2007) 1249−1255.

[5] S.A. Ranadive, J.D. Pipkin, S.A. Varia, N.H. Chang, E.P. Barry, M. Porubcan, S.E. Unger, T.J. McCormick, Formation, isolation and identification of oligomers of aztreonam, Eur. J. Pharm. Sci. 3 (1995) 281−291.

[6] P. Fyhr, C. Högström, A preformulation study on the kinetics of the racemization of ropivacaine hydrochloride, Acta Pharm. Suecica 25 (1988) 121−132.

ANSWERS TO LEARNING QUESTIONS AND PROBLEMS

Question 2.1

There are two main reasons for this: 1) In general, the mobile phase contains organic solvents that decrease the drug affinity for the cyclo-dextrin cavity. 2) The drug molecules bound within the complex are in a very dynamic equilibrium with free drug molecules in the solution and are very rapidly released upon dilution at the time the sample enters the HPLC column. However, it is possible to affect the drug retention time by the addition of cyclodextrin to an aqueous mobile phase (thus preventing drug release upon dilution).

Question 3.1

Both profiles can be explained by Eq. 3.6, that is, specific acid (k_H) and solvent (k_0) catalyzed hydrolysis of the unionized form, and solvent (k'_0) and specific base (k'_{OH}) catalyzed hydrolysis of the ionized form is expressed:

$$k_{obs} = k_H[H^+]f_{AH} + k_0f_{AH} + k'_0f_{A^-} + k'_{OH}[OH^-]f_{A^-}$$

However, due to intramolecular catalysis, k_0 is smaller than k'_0 for aspirin (the acetoxy moiety in *ortho* position), while no intramolecular catalysis is possible in the case of *p*-acetoxybenzoate. Consequently, k_0 is larger than k'_0 when the acetoxy moiety is in the *para* position.

Question 3.2

As shown in the following figure, the first step of the reaction is the forma-tion of the aziridinium ring, which is followed by the nucleophilic attack of water:

Aziridinium ring

The rate equation for this first step is:

$$-\frac{d[\text{Chlorambucil}]}{dt} = k_1[\text{Chlorambucil}] - k_{-1}[\text{Aziridinium ring}][\text{Cl}^-]$$

Thus, the equilibrium shifts toward the left with increasing chloride concentration, and the concentration of the cyclic intermediate (the aziridinium ring) decreases. The next step is the nucleophilic attack of water on the intermediate:

$$-\frac{d[\text{Aziridinium ring}]}{dt} = k_{-1}[\text{Aziridiniusm ring}][\text{Cl}^-]$$
$$+ k_2'[\text{Aziridinium ring}][\text{H}_2\text{O}] - k_1[\text{Chlorambucil}]$$

Since the reaction takes place in an aqueous solution, the concentration of water will remain essentially constant or $k_2[\text{H}_2\text{O}] \approx k_2'$. Furthermore, it can be assumed that the concentration of the aziridinium intermediate will remain constant (see Chapter2, section 2.6.4 Steady-state approximation):

$$-\frac{d[\text{Aziridinium ring}]}{dt} = 0 = k_{-1}[\text{Aziridiniusm ring}][\text{Cl}^-]$$
$$+ k_2'[\text{Aziridinium ring}] - k_1[\text{Chlorambucil}]$$

$$[\text{Aziridinium ring}] = \frac{k_1}{k_{-1}[\text{Cl}^-] + k_2'}[\text{Chlorambucil}]$$

The rate equation for formation of the product is:

$$\frac{d[\text{Product}]}{dt} = k_2[\text{Aziridinium ring}][\text{H}_2\text{O}] = k_2'[\text{Aziridinium ring}]$$

or

$$\frac{d[\text{Product}]}{dt} = \frac{k_1 k_2'}{k_{-1}[\text{Cl}^-] + k_2'}[\text{Chlorambucil}] = k_{\text{obs}}[\text{Chlorambucil}]$$

$$k_{\text{obs}} = \frac{k_1 k_2'}{k_{-1}[\text{Cl}^-] + k_2'}$$

The value of k_{obs} will decrease with increasing chloride concentration ($[\text{Cl}^-]$).

Question 3.3

Apparently, COL-3 is susceptible to oxidative degradation. Ascorbic acid, sodium bisulfite, and EDTA (edetic acid or its sodium salt disodium edetate) are antioxidants (see section 3.2.5). Ascorbic acid and sodium bisulfite protect COL-3 by being reducing agents (have lower reduction potentials than COL-3 and, thus, are more susceptible to oxidation than COL-3). EDTA is a chelating agent that inactivates oxidative catalysis by metal ions. In general, chelating agents are not antioxidants as such, but are used in combination with antioxidants (such as reduction agents) to improve their efficacy.

Question 3.4

Prostaglandin B_2 has conjugated double bonds. In general, conjugated double bonds are more stable than isolated double bonds.

Prostaglandin $A_2 \rightarrow$ prostaglandin B_2 is a type of isomerization.

Question 3.5

Methanol has just one OH group and, thus, terminates the polymerization. Formation of a penicillin dimer is the first step in the penicillin polymerization, then the trimer is formed followed by the tetramer, the pentamer and so on. Thus, the penicillin polymer consists of polymers of different chain lengths. It is difficult to monitor formation of all the different polymer chain lengths. The investigators selected to monitor the pentamer concentration. In the beginning the concentrations of dimers and trimers are low but but it increases with time. As the concentration of the trimer increases the rate of the tetramer formation increases resulting in positive deviation.

Question 5.1

An intermolecular reaction is reaction between molecules while an intramolecular reaction is a reaction within a molecule (e.g., intramolecular thiol/disulfide exchange reactions in proteins).

Intermolecular catalysis is the catalysis of a chemical reaction in one molecule through involvement of another molecule or ion (e.g., buffer catalysis or general acid/base catalysis). Intramolecular catalysis is a catalysis of a chemical reaction at one site of a molecule through involvement of another catalytic group within the same molecule (e.g., intramolecular catalysis of aspirin hydrolysis in Fig. 3.5).

ANSWERS TO PROBLEMS IN CHAPTER 8:

8.1:

The results are arranged (see table) and plotted according to Eq. 2.52:

$$t = \frac{1}{(k_f + k_r)} \ln \frac{[A]_0 - [A]_{eq}}{[A] - [A]_{eq}}$$

$$\ln \frac{100 - 50}{86.6 - 50} = \ln \frac{50}{36.6} = 0.312$$

$$\ln \frac{100 - 50}{76.8 - 50} = \ln \frac{50}{26.8} = 0.624$$

and so on. . .

Time (min)	% (R)-Oxazepam	$\ln \frac{[A]_0 - [A]_{eq}}{[A] - [A]_{eq}}$
15	86.6	0.312
30	76.8	0.624
45	69.6	0.903
60	64.4	1.245

Racemization: $k_f = k_r$, $K = 1.00$, and $[A]_{eq} = [B]_{eq} = 50\%$

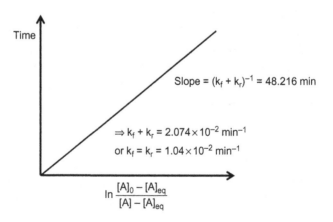

$$t_{90} = \frac{1}{(k_f + k_r)} \times \ln \frac{100 - 50}{90 - 50} = 48.216 \times \ln 1.25 = 10.8 \text{ min}$$

8.2:

We will apply Eq. 2.70 to solve this problem:

$$A \xrightarrow{k_A} B \xrightarrow{k_B} C \qquad [B] = \frac{k_A[A]_0}{(k_B - k_A)}(e^{-k_A t} - e^{-k_B t}),$$

but after some time virtually all A has degraded to form B (see the figure that follows in which the Y-axis is in a common log scale):

At 40 hours, virtually all A (i.e., PGE_2) has been converted into B (i.e., PGA_2), and Eq. 2.70 can be simplified to:

$$[B]' = \frac{k_A[A]_0}{(k_A - k_B)}(e^{-k_B t})$$

From 40 hours:

$$\ln[B]' = \ln\left(\frac{k_A[A]_0}{(k_A - k_B)}\right) - k_B \times t$$

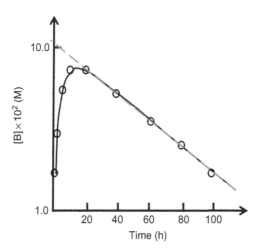

From 0 to 20 hours, we can use the following equation to calculate k_A:

$$[B]' - [B] = \frac{k_A[A]_0}{(k_A - k_B)}(e^{-k_A t})$$

or

$$\ln \left([B]' - [B]\right) = \ln \left(\frac{k_A[A]_0}{(k_A - k_B)}\right) - k_A \times t$$

Time (h)	[B] 10^2 (M)	ln ([B] 10^2)	[B]' 10^2 (M)	([B]' − [B]) 10^2 (M)	ln([B]' − [B])
1	1.71		10.8682	9.1582	−2.3905
2	3.10		10.6689	7.5689	−2.5811
5	5.82		10.0929	4.2729	−3.1529
10	7.55		9.2011	1.6511	−4.1037
20	7.41		7.6469	0.2369	−6.0453
40	5.28	−2.941	5.2818		−
60	3.65	−3.310			
80	2.52	−3.681			
100	1.74	−4.051			

t from 40 to 100 h:

$$\text{Slope} = -k_B = -1.8505 \times 10^{-2} h^{-1} \Rightarrow k_B = 1.85 \times 10^{-2} h^{-1}$$

$$\ln \left(\frac{k_A[A]_0}{(k_A - k_B)}\right) = \text{Intercept} = -2.2004 \Rightarrow e^{-2.2004} = 0.1108 \text{ M}$$

t from 1 to 20 h:

$$\text{Slope} = -k_A = -0.1923 \text{ h}^{-1} \Rightarrow k_A = 0.192 \text{ h}^{-1}$$

$$\ln \left(\frac{k_A[A]_0}{(k_A - k_B)}\right) = \text{Intercept} = -2.1933 \Rightarrow e^{-2.1933} = 0.1115 \text{ M}$$

The shelf-life of PGE_2 is calculated from Eq. 2.19:

$$t_{90} = \frac{0.105}{k_A} = \frac{0.105}{0.192 \text{ h}^{-1}} = 0.55 \text{ h}$$

8.3:
The problem can be solved by a nonlinear fit of the experimental data to Eq. 2.174. However, here we use the Lineweaver-Burk plot (Eq. 2.175), where $(k_f - k_{obs})^{-1}$ *versus* $([Tris]_T)^{-1}$ will give a straight line from which k_c can be obtained from the intercept and $K_{1:1}$ from the slope:

$$\frac{1}{k_f - k_{obs}} = \frac{1}{K_{1:1} \cdot (k_f - k_c)} \cdot \frac{1}{[CD]_T} + \frac{1}{k_f - k_c}$$
$$= \frac{1}{K_{1:1} \cdot (k_f - k_c)} \cdot \frac{1}{[Tris]_T} + \frac{1}{k_f - k_c}$$

[Tris] (M)	$[Tris]^{-1}$ (M^{-1})	k_{obs} (min^{-1})	$\frac{1}{k_f - k_{obs}}$
0.000	–	0.4234	–
0.050	20.00	0.2856	7.2569
0.125	8.00	0.2482	5.7078
0.175	5.71	0.2251	5.0429
0.250	4.00	0.2137	4.7687
0.500	2.00	0.2044	4.5662

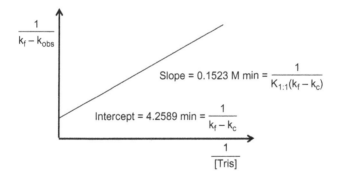

$K_{1:1}$ = Intercept÷Slope = 4.2589 min÷0.1523 M min = 28.0 M^{-1}

k_f = 0.4234 min^{-1} (from the previous table at [Tris] = 0.000)

$$4.2589 = \frac{1}{0.4234 - k_c} \Rightarrow k_c = 0.1886 \text{ min}^{-1}$$
$$192.77 \text{ min} = (1.49 \times 10^{-2} - k_c)^{-1} \Rightarrow k_c = 9.71 \times 10^{-3} \text{ min}^{-1}$$

$k_f = 0.42 \text{ min}^{-1}$, $k_c = 0.19 \text{ min}^{-1}$ and $K_{1:1} = 28.0 \text{ M}^{-1}$ at pH 8.0 and 55°C

8.4:
A:

pH	k_{obs} (h^{-1})	$\log k_{obs}$
1.00	15.31×10^{-2}	-0.815
1.50	6.166×10^{-2}	-1.21
2.00	3.236×10^{-2}	-1.49
2.50	1.905×10^{-2}	-1.72
3.00	1.023×10^{-2}	-1.99
3.50	0.447×10^{-2}	-2.35
4.00	0.158×10^{-2}	-2.80
5.00	0.170×10^{-2}	-2.77
6.00	0.158×10^{-2}	-2.80
7.00	1.445×10^{-2}	-1.84
7.50	2.140×10^{-2}	-1.67
8.00	3.236×10^{-2}	-1.49
9.00	5.012×10^{-2}	-1.30
10.00	32.36×10^{-2}	-0.490

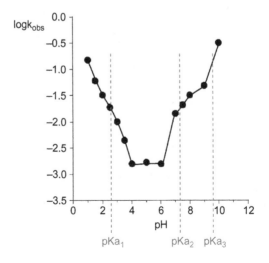

B:
Each of the four ionic species can, in theory, display specific acid–catalyzed (k_H), uncatalyzed (k_0), and specific base catalyzed (k_{OH})

degradation. However, the pH-rate profile indicates that some of these do not occur in the pH interval in which given ionic species are present in the degradation media. Only one of the four ionic forms displays all three types of degradation (see Chapter 3, Section 3.1.4):

$$k_{obs} = k_H[H^+]f_{AH_3} + k'_H[H^+]f_{AH_2} + k'_0 f_{AH_2} + k'_{OH}[H^+]f_{AH_2}$$
$$+ k''_{OH}[OH^-]f_{AH} + k'''_{OH}[OH^-]f_A$$

$$-\frac{d[A]_T}{dt} = k_{obs}[A]_T$$

$$[A]_T = [AH_3] + [AH_2] + [AH] + [A]$$

$$f_{AH_3} = \frac{[H^+]^3}{[H^+]^3 + [H^+]^2 K_{a1} + [H^+]K_{a1}K_{a2} + K_{a1}K_{a2}K_{a3}}$$

$$f_{AH_2} = \frac{[H^+]^2 K_{a1}}{[H^+]^3 + [H^+]^2 K_{a1} + [H^+]K_{a1}K_{a2} + K_{a1}K_{a2}K_{a3}}$$

$$f_{AH} = \frac{[H^+]K_{a1}K_{a2}}{[H^+]^3 + [H^+]^2 K_{a1} + [H^+]K_{a1}K_{a2} + K_{a1}K_{a2}K_{a3}}$$

$$f_A = \frac{K_{a1}K_{a2}K_{a3}}{[H^+]^3 + [H^+]^2 K_{a1} + [H^+]K_{a1}K_{a2} + K_{a1}K_{a2}K_{a3}}$$

At pH = 1.0:

$f_{AH_3} \approx 1.00$ and, thus, $k_{obs} \approx k_H[H^+] \times 1.00 = 0.1531\ h^{-1}$. $[H^+] = 10^{-1}\ M$

$$k_H = \frac{0.1531\ h^{-1}}{10^{-1}M} = 1.53\ M^{-1}h^{-1}$$

At pH = 5.0:

Relatively flat bottom and $k_{obs} = 0.170 \times 10^{-2}\ h^{-1}$. $f_{AH_2} \approx 1.00$ and, thus, $k_{obs} = k_0' \times 1.00 \Rightarrow k_0' = 0.170 \times 10^{-2} h^{-1}$

At pH = 3.0:

$$f_{AH_3} = \frac{[H^+]^3}{[H^+]^3 + [H^+]^2 K_{a1} + [H^+]K_{a1}K_{a2} + K_{a1}K_{a2}K_{a3}}$$

$$= \frac{(10^{-3})^3}{(10^{-3})^3 + (10^{-3})^2 \times 10^{-2.97} + (10^{-3}) \times 10^{-2.97} \times 10^{-7.28} + 10^{-2.97} \times 10^{-7.28} \times 10^{-9.65}}$$

$$= \frac{10^{-9}}{2.0716 \times 10^{-9}} = 0.483$$

$$f_{AH_2} \approx 0.517$$

$$k_{obs} = 1.023 \times 10^{-2} = k_H[H^+]f_{AH_3} + k_H'[H^+]f_{AH_2} + k_0'f_{AH_2} \Rightarrow$$

$$1.023 \times 10^{-2}h^{-1} = 1.53\ M^{-1}h^{-1} \times 10^{-3}M \times 0.483$$
$$+ k_H' \times 10^{-3}M \times 0.517 + 0.170 \times 10^{-2}h^{-1} \times 0.517$$

$$1.023 \times 10^{-2}h^{-1} = 7.543 \times 10^{-4}h^{-1} + k_H' \times 0.517 \times 10^{-3}M$$
$$+ 8.789 \times 10^{-4}h^{-1}$$

$$k_H' = 16.6\ M^{-1}h^{-1}$$

At pH = 10.0:

Here we have to assume that $f_A \approx 1.00$ and $k_{obs} \approx k'''_{OH}[OH^-]f_A = k'''_{OH} \times 10^{-(13.6-10.0)} \times 1.000.3236\,h^{-1} = k'''_{OH} \times 10^{-3.6}M \Rightarrow k'''_{OH} \approx 1300\,M^{-1}h^{-1}$. However, this value is not very accurate since pK_{a3} is 9.65, and consequently $f_A = 0.69$ and $f_{AH} = 0.31$. Thus, it is not correct to completely ignore the contribution of k''_{OH} at pH 10.0.

At pH = 9.0:

$$f_A = \frac{K_{a1}K_{a2}K_{a3}}{[H^+]^3 + [H^+]^2K_{a1} + [H^+]K_{a1}K_{a2} + K_{a1}K_{a2}K_{a3}}$$

$$= \frac{10^{-2.97} \times 10^{-7.28} \times 10^{-9.65}}{(10^{-9})^3 + (10^{-9})^2 \times 10^{-2.97} + (10^{-9}) \times 10^{-2.97} \times 10^{-7.28} + 10^{-2.97} \times 10^{-7.28} \times 10^{-9.65}}$$

$$= \frac{1.2589 \times 10^{-20}}{6.989 \times 10^{-20}} = 0.18$$

$$f_{AH} \approx 0.82$$

$$k_{obs} = k''_{OH}[OH^-]f_{AH} + k'''_{OH}[OH^-]f_A \Rightarrow$$

$$5.012 \times 10^{-2}h^{-1} \approx k''_{OH} \times 10^{-4.6}M \times 0.82 + 1300\,M^{-1}h^{-1} \times 10^{-4.6}M \times 0.18$$

$$= k''_{OH} \times 2.060 \times 10^{-5}M + 5.878 \times 10^{-3}h^{-1}$$
$$k''_{OH} = 2150\,M^{-1}h^{-1}$$

There is some error in this value, since the value of k'''_{OH} is somewhat inaccurate.

At pH = 7.0:

$$f_{AH_2} = \frac{[H^+]^2K_{a1}}{[H^+]^3 + [H^+]^2K_{a1} + [H^+]K_{a1}K_{a2} + K_{a1}K_{a2}K_{a3}}$$

$$= \frac{(10^{-7})^2 \times 10^{-2.97}}{(10^{-7})^3 + (10^{-7})^2 \times 10^{-2.97} + (10^{-7}) \times 10^{-2.97} \times 10^{-7.28} + 10^{-2.97} \times 10^{-7.28} \times 10^{-9.65}}$$

$$= \frac{1.0715 \times 10^{-17}}{1.6352 \times 10^{-17}} = 0.655$$

$$f_{AH} = 0.345$$

$$k_{obs} = k'_0 f_{AH_2} + k'_{OH}[H^+]f_{AH_2} + k''_{OH}[OH^-]f_{AH} \Rightarrow$$

$$1.445 \times 10^{-2} h^{-1} = 0.170 \times 10^{-2} h^{-1} \times 0.655 + k'_{OH} \times 10^{-7} M \times 0.655$$
$$+ 2150 \ M^{-1} h^{-1} \times 10^{-7} M \times 0.345$$

$$1.445 \times 10^{-2} h^{-1} = 1.1135 \times 10^{-3} h^{-1} + k'_{OH} \times 6.55 \times 10^{-8} M$$
$$+ 7.4175 \times 10^{-5} h^{-1}$$

$$k'_{OH} = 2.02 \times 10^5 M^{-1} h^{-1}$$

The equation for the observed rate constant for the degradation of amoxicillin in an aqueous solution at 35°C and I = 0.5 is:

$$k_{obs} = 1.53 \ M^{-1} h^{-1} [H^+] f_{AH_3} + 16.6 \ M^{-1} h^{-1} [H^+] f_{AH_2}$$
$$+ 0.170 \times 10^{-2} h^{-1} f_{AH_2} + 2.02 \times 10^5 M^{-1} h^{-1} [H^+] f_{AH_2}$$
$$+ 2150 \ M^{-1} h^{-1} [OH^-] f_{AH} + 1300 \ M^{-1} h^{-1} [OH^-] f_A$$

C:
We will use Eqs. 2.100, 2.101, 2.113, and 2.125 to 2.128 to solve this problem.

According to $k = PZe^{-\frac{E_a}{RT}}$ (Eq. 2.100) and $k = Ae^{-\frac{E_a}{RT}}$ (Eq. 2.101, Arrhenius equation), $A = P \times Z$.

Furthermore, $P = e^{\frac{\Delta S^{\neq}}{R}}$ (Eq. 2.127) and $Z = \dfrac{RT}{Nh}$ (Eq. 2.126).

Using the Arrhenius equation, we can calculate the value of A (the frequency factor):

$$1.70 \times 10^{-3} h^{-1} = A \times e^{-\frac{18100 \ cal \ mol^{-1}}{1.9872 \ cal \ mol^{-1} K^{-1} \times 308 \ K}} \Rightarrow A = 1.1845964 \cdot 10^{10} h^{-1}$$

$$A = e^{\frac{\Delta S^{\neq}}{R}} \times \frac{R \times T}{N \times h}$$

$$1.1845964 \times 10^{10} h^{-1}$$

$$= e^{\frac{\Delta S^{\neq}}{R}} \times \frac{8.3143 \times 10^{7} erg\,mol^{-1} K^{-1} \times 308\,K \times 60\,s\,min^{-1} \times 60\,min\,h^{-1}}{6.022 \times 10^{23} mol^{-1} \times 6.6262 \times 10^{-27} erg\,s}$$

$$\Rightarrow P = e^{\frac{\Delta S^{\neq}}{R}} = 5.1274 \times 10^{-6} \Rightarrow \Delta S^{\neq}/R = -14,483 \Rightarrow$$

$\Delta S^{\neq} = -28.8 \; cal\;mol^{-1} \quad K^{-1} = -120\;J\;mol^{-1}\;K^{-1}, \quad$ and $\quad P = 5.12 \times 10^{-6}$

$\Delta H^{\neq} \approx E_a = 18.100 \; cal/mol$

$\Delta G^{\neq} = \Delta H^{\neq} - T \times \Delta S^{\neq} = 18100 - 308\,(-28.8) = 26.970 \; cal/mol = 27.0 \; kcal/mol = 113 \; kJ/mol$

8.5:

Glucose catalyzes the degradation through the formation of an amox-icillin/glucose complex:

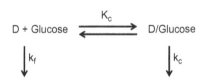

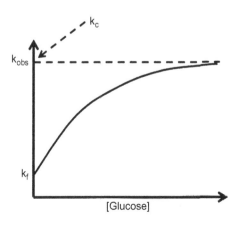

$$\frac{1}{k_f - k_{obs}} = \frac{1}{K_{1:1} \cdot (k_f - k_c)} \cdot \frac{1}{[\text{Glucose}]_T} + \frac{1}{k_f - k_c}$$

Glucose (% w/v)	Glucose (mol/liter)	$[\text{Glucose}]^{-1}\ M^{-1}$	k_{obs} (min^{-1})	$\dfrac{1}{k_f - k_{obs}}$
0	0.000	–	$2.38\ 10^{-2}$	–
5	0.278	3.60	$8.18\ 10^{-2}$	-17.24
10	0.556	1.80	$13.30\ 10^{-2}$	-9.158

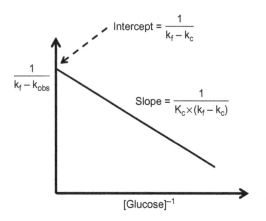

$$\text{Intercept} = -1.076\ \text{min} \Rightarrow k_f - k_c = -0.9294\ \text{min}^{-1}$$
$$\Rightarrow k_c = k_f + 0.9294 = 0.953\ \text{min}^{-1}$$
$$K_{1:1} = \text{Intercept} \div \text{Slope} = -1.076\ \text{min} \div -4.49\ \text{M min} = 0.24\ \text{M}^{-1}$$

$k_f = 2.38\ 10^{-2}\text{min}^{-1}$, $k_c = 0.953\ \text{min}^{-1}$, and $K_{1:1} = 0.24\ \text{M}^{-1}$
at pH 7.4 and 75°C

8.6:
Here, we estimate the rate constants from the pH-rate profile. First we determine the equation for k_{obs} based on the possible ionization species and the shape of the pH-rate profile:

$$k_{obs} = k_H[\text{H}^+]f_{\text{H}_2\text{A}} + k_0 f_{\text{H}_2\text{A}} + k_{OH}[\text{OH}^-]f_{\text{H}_2\text{A}} + k'_{OH}[\text{OH}^-]f_{\text{HA}^-}$$
$$+ k''_{OH}[\text{OH}^-]f_{\text{A}^{2-}}$$

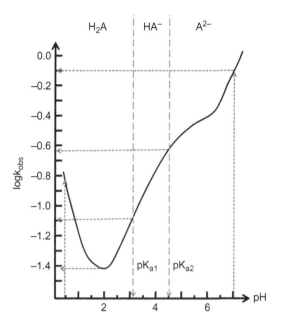

$$f_{H_2A} = \frac{[H^+]^2}{[H^+]^2 + [H^+]K_{a1} + K_{a1}K_{a2}} \qquad f_{HA} = \frac{[H^+]K_{a1}}{[H^+]^2 + [H^+]K_{a1} + K_{a1}K_{a2}}$$

$$f_A = \frac{K_{a1}K_{a2}}{[H^+]^2 + [H^+]K_{a1} + K_{a1}K_{a2}}$$

Then we estimate the individual rate constants:

$pH = 7.0$: $f_{H_2A} = 4.5 \times 10^{-7} \approx 0.00$ $f_{HA} = 0.002$ $f_A = 1.00$

$k_{obs} = k''_{OH}[OH^-]f_{A^{2-}}$ or $0.79 = k''_{OH} \times 5.55 \times 10^{-6} \times 1.00$

$k''_{OH} \approx 1.4 \times 10^5 \, M^{-1}h^{-1}$

$pH = 4.5$: $f_{H_2A} \approx 0.00$ $f_{HA} = 0.5$ $f_A = 0.5$

$k_{obs} = k'_{OH}[OH^-]f_{HA^-} + k''_{OH}[OH^-]f_{A^{2-}}$ $k_{obs} = 10^{-0.63} = 0.23 \, h^{-1}$ or

$0.23 = k'_{OH} \times 10^{-7.95} \times 0.50 + 1.4 \times 10^5 \times 10^{-7.95} \times 0.50$

$k'_{OH} \approx 4.1 \, 10^7 \, M^{-1}h^{-1}$

$pH = 3.1$: $f_{H_2A} = 0.5$ $f_{HA} = 0.5$ $f_A \approx 0.00$

$k_{obs} = k_{OH}[OH^-]f_{H_2A} + k'_{OH}[OH^-]f_{HA^-}$ $k_{obs} = 10^{-1.1} = 0.08\,h^{-1}$

$0.08 = k_{OH} \times 10^{-9.31} \times 0.50 + 4.1 \times 10^7 \times 10^{-9.31} \times 0.50$

$k_{OH} \approx 2.9\,10^8\,M^{-1}h^{-1}$

$pH = 0.5$: $f_{H_2A} = 1.00$ $f_{HA} \approx 0.00$ $f_A \approx 0.00$

$k_{obs} = k_H[H^+]f_{H_2A}$ $k_{obs} = 10^{-0.83} = 0.15\,h^{-1}$

$0.15 = k_H \times 10^{-0.5} \times 1.00$ $k_H \approx 0.5\,M^{-1}h^{-1}$

$pH = 2.0$: $f_{H_2A} = 0.93$ $f_{HA} = 0.07$ $f_A \approx 0.00$

$k_{obs} = k_H[H^+]f_{H_2A} + k_0 f_{H_2A} + k_{OH}[OH^-]f_{H_2A} + k'_{OH}[OH^-]f_{HA^-}$

$k_{obs} = 10^{-1.4} = 0.04\,h^{-1}$

$0.04 = 0.5 \times 10^{-2} \times 0.93 + k_0 \times 0.93 + 2.9 \times 10^8 \times 10^{-10.45} \times 0.93$
$+ 4.1 \times 10^7 \times 10^{-10.45} \times 0.07$

$0.04 = 4.65 \times 10^{-3} + k_0 \times 0.93 + 9.57 \times 10^{-3} + 1.01 \times 10^{-4}$
$k_0 \approx 0.03\,h^{-1}$

8.7:

Formation of the dimer (D) is probably a second-order reaction in which two molecules of aztreonam collide to form the dimer $(A + A \rightarrow D)$, see Eqs. 2.26, 2.30, and 2.31:

$$\frac{d[D]}{dt} = k_2[A]^2 \ \ \text{or} \ \ t = \frac{1}{k_2}\left(\frac{1}{[A]} - \frac{1}{[A]_0}\right) \ \text{and} \ \ t_{\frac{1}{2}} = \frac{1}{k_2[A]_0}.$$

Formation of the trimer (T) could be a third-order reaction $(A + A + A \rightarrow D)$:

$$\frac{d[T]}{dt} = k_3[A]^3 \text{ or } t = \frac{1}{2k_3}\left(\frac{1}{[A]^2} - \frac{1}{[A]_0^2}\right) \text{ and } t_{\frac{1}{2}} = \frac{1}{2k_3[A]_0^2}.$$

It is also possible that the trimer is formed when a dimer reacts with a monomer, a tetramer is formed when two dimers react and so on. The figure shows that the rate of formation of P $(d[P]/dt)$ increases rapidly with increasing aztreonam concentration. However, the rate equations show that the rate of dimer formation is proportional to the second power and the formation rate of the trimer is proportional to the third power of the aztreonam concentration and, thus, the increase is perhaps less than expected. In fact, it has been shown that the value of the observed second-order rate constant, k_2, decreases with increasing aztreonam concentration and that the stability of aztreonam cannot be predicted from its stability in dilute solutions due to differences in its degradation mechanism [1]. One would assume that the dimer formation would dominate at a low aztreonam concentration, but that the rate of formation of the trimer and higher order oligomers would rapidly increase with increasing initial aztreonam concentration leading to changes in the degradation mechanism.

8.8:

Use the Q_{10} method (see Chapter 2, section 2.7.1) to estimate k_{obs} at 25°C. The value of Q_{10} is between 2 and 4. Thus, the estimated maximum value ($Q_{10} = 2$) of k_{obs} at 25°C will be $1 \times 10^{-6} s^{-1}$ (min. k_{obs} value ($Q_{10} = 4$) at 25°C is $0.5 \times 10^{-6} s^{-1}$). The zero-order rate constant (k_0) will then be:

$$k_0 = k_{obs} \times S_0 = 1 \times 10^{-6}s^{-1} \times 10 \text{ mg/ml} = 1 \times 10^{-5} \frac{mg}{s \, ml}$$

$$t_{90} = \frac{0.10 \, [Drug]_{total}}{k_0} = \frac{0.10 \times 25 \frac{mg}{ml}}{1 \times 10^{-5} \frac{mg}{s \, ml}} = 2.50 \times 10^5 s = 69 \text{ h} = 2.9 \text{ days}$$

This is shelf-life a bit too short as most antibiotic therapies last for about one week or more. We should be able to at least double the shelf-life (assuming a Q_{10} of at least 2) by lowering the storage temperature by 10°C. Thus, the shelf-life will be at least 5.8 days at 15°C and 12 days at 5°C. Greater shelf-life enhancement will be observed if Q_{10} is greater than 2 and/or if the solubility lowers with decreasing temperature.

If Q_{10} is 4, then $t_{90} = 4 \times 4 \times 2.9 = 46$ days at 5°C. It can be assumed that t_{90} of the antibiotic mixture will never exceed a few months, even if the solubility will be somewhat lower at 5°C than at 25°C. Thus, this antibiotic suspension will never be distributed as a ready-to-use antibiotic formulation. It will be distributed as a powder for oral suspension. The common shelf-life of such powders is three years, but is only between one and two weeks after reconstitution as an oral suspension.

8.9:
Eq. 2.52 is applied to solve this problem:

$$t = \frac{1}{(k_1 + k_{-1})} \times \ln \frac{[A]_0 - [A]_{Eq}}{[A] - [A]_{Eq}} \quad \text{or} \quad \ln \frac{[A]_0 - [A]_{Eq}}{[A] - [A]_{Eq}} = (k_1 + k_{-1}) \times t$$

Racemization and, thus, $K = 1.00$ and $[A]_{Eq} = 50$.

Time (days)	% Ropivacaine (i.e. the S-form)	$A - A_{Eq}$	$\ln \dfrac{[A]_0 - [A]_{Eq}}{[A] - [A]_{Eq}}$
1.0	94.6	44.6	0.114
2.5	84.3	34.3	0.377
5.0	75.9	25.9	0.658
10	62.2	12.2	1.411
15	56.2	6.2	2.087

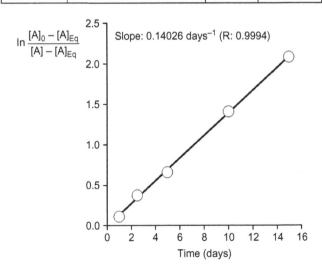

$k_1 + k_{-1} = 0.14026\,\text{days}^{-1}$ $K_{Eq} = 1.00$ and, thus, $k_1 = k_{-1} \Rightarrow k_1 = k_{-1} = 7.01 \times 10^{-2}\,\text{days}^{-1}$

$$t_{90}: \ln\frac{100-50}{90-50} = 0.14026 \times t_{90} \Rightarrow t_{90} = 1.59\ \text{days}.$$

8.10:

pH	k_{obs} (h^{-1})	logk_{obs}
1.0	4.53×10^{-5}	−4.344
2.0	3.60×10^{-6}	−5.444
3.0	2.27×10^{-7}	−6.644
3.7	5.71×10^{-8}	−7.243
4.0	1.14×10^{-7}	−6.943
5.0	1.14×10^{-6}	−5.943
6.0	7.18×10^{-6}	−5.144
7.0	7.18×10^{-5}	−4.144
8.0	3.60×10^{-4}	−3.444
9.0	1.80×10^{-3}	−2.745
10.0	1.80×10^{-2}	−1.745
11.0	1.80×10^{-1}	−0.745

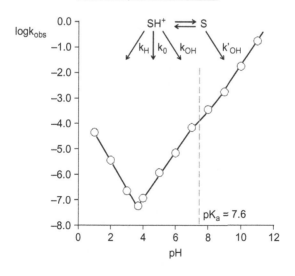

$$k_{obs} = k_H[H^+]f_{SH} + k_0f_{SH} + k_{OH}[OH^-]f_{SH} + k'_{OH}[OH^-]f_S$$

At pH = 2.0: $k_{obs} = k_H[H^+]f_{SH}$ or $3.60 \times 10^{-6}\ h^{-1}$
$$= k_H \times 10^{-2} \times 1.00   k_H = 3.60 \times 10^{-4}\ M^{-1}\ h^{-1}$$

At pH = 6.0: $k_{obs} = k_{OH}[OH^-]f_{SH}$ or $7.18 \times 10^{-6}\ h^{-1}$
$$= k_{OH} \times 10^{-(14-6)} \times 1.00   k_{OH} = 718\ M^{-1}h^{-1}$$

At pH = 10.0: $k_{obs} = k'_{OH}[OH^-]f_S$ or $1.80 \times 10^{-2}\ h^{-1}$
$$= k_{OH} \times 10^{-(14-10)} \times 1.00   k'_{OH} = 180\ M^{-1}h^{-1}$$

At pH = 3.7: $k_{obs} = k_H[H^+]f_{SH} + k_0f_{SH} + k_{OH}[OH^-]f_{SH}$ or

$$5.71 \times 10^{-8} = 3.60 \times 10^{-4} \times 10^{-3.7} \times 1.00 + k_0 \times 1.00$$
$$+ 718 \times 10^{-(14.0-3.7)} \times 1.00$$

$$5.71 \times 10^{-8} = 7.183 \times 10^{-8} + k_0 + 3.560 \times 10^{-8}\ (k_0 < 0) \Rightarrow k_0 \approx 0\ h^{-1}$$

or $k_{obs} = 3.60 \times 10^{-4}[H^+]f_{SH} + 718[OH^-]f_{SH} + 180[OH^-]f_S$

However, there are two parallel reactions (see Chapter 2, Section 2.6.2) at pH >3 (i.e., hydrolysis and isomerization) and the relative contribution can be calculated from the relative concentration of the product according to Eqs. 2.61 and 2.62. For the protonated form (SH$^+$) we have:

$$k_{HY} = k_{OH}\frac{[A]}{[A] + [B]} = 718 \times 0.96 = 689\ M^{-1}h^{-1}$$

$$k_{IS} = k_{OH}\frac{[A]}{[A] + [B]} = 718 \times 0.04 = 29\ M^{-1}h^{-1}$$

For the uncharged drug (S) we have:

$$k'_{HY} = k'_{OH} \frac{[A]}{[A] + [B]} = 180 \times 0.72 = 130 \text{ M}^{-1}\text{h}^{-1}$$

$$k'_{IS} = k'_{OH} \frac{[A]}{[A] + [B]} = 180 \times 0.28 = 50 \text{ M}^{-1}\text{h}^{-1}$$

Thus, the more correct equation for the observed rate constant is

$$k_{obs} = k_H[H^+]f_{SH} + k_{HY}[OH^-]f_{SH} + k_{IS}[OH^-]f_{SH}$$
$$+ k'_{HY}[OH^-]f_S + k'_{IS}[OH^-]f_S$$

or $k_{obs} = k_H[H^+]f_{SH} + (k_{HY} + k_{IS})[OH^-]f_{SH} + (k'_{HY} + k'_{IS})[OH^-]f_S$

8.11:

Isotonic (0.9% w/v) NaCl (molecular weight 58.44 g/mol) solution contains:

$$[Na^+] = [Cl^-] = 9.0/55.44 = 0.162 \text{ mol/liter}$$
$$I = \tfrac{1}{2}(0.162 \cdot (+1)^2 + 0.162 \cdot (-1)^2) = 0.16 \text{ mol/liter} \approx 0.16 \text{ mol/Kg}$$

We will apply Eq. 2.158:

$$\log k_{obs} = \log k_0 + 1.02 z_A z_B \frac{\sqrt{I}}{1 + \sqrt{I}} = \log k_0 + \text{Slope} \times \frac{\sqrt{I}}{1 + \sqrt{I}}$$

I (mol/liter)	$\sqrt{I}$	$\frac{\sqrt{I}}{1+\sqrt{I}}$	k_{obs} (s^{-1})	$\log k_{obs}$
0.10	0.316	0.240	3.16×10^{-3}	-2.500
0.25	0.500	0.333	7.94×10^{-3}	-2.100
0.31	0.557	0.358	8.51×10^{-3}	-2.070
0.00	0.000	0.000	$k_0 = 3.89 \times 10^{-4}$	$\log k_0 = -3.410$
0.16	0.400	0.286	$k_{0.16} = 4.81 \times 10^{-3}$	$\log k_{0.16} = -2.318$

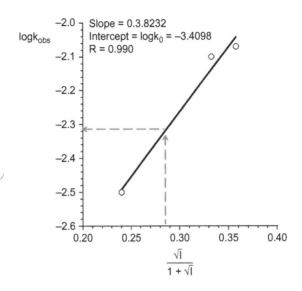

Eq. 2.19 is applied to calculate t_{90}:

$$At\ I = 0.00: \quad t_{90} = \frac{0.105}{k_0} = \frac{0.105}{3.89 \times 10^{-4} s^{-1}} = 270\ s = 4.5\ minutes$$

$$At\ I = 0.16: \quad t_{90} = \frac{0.105}{k_{0.16}} = \frac{0.105}{4.81 \times 10^{-3} s^{-1}} = 22\ s = 0.4\ minutes$$

The pH-rate profile for the apaziquone degradation on aqueous solution is V-shaped, displaying maximum stability at pH 8.6. At this pH, apaziquone is over 10,000 times more stable than at pH 4.0 (t_{90} at pH 8.6 and 25°C is about 3.8 days) [2].

8.12:

Aspirin: $k_{obs} = k_H[H^+]f_{AH} + k_0 f_{AH} + k_0' f_{A^-} + k_{OH}'[OH^-]f_{A^-}$

Methylsalicylate (at pH below 10): $k_{obs} = k_H[H^+] + k_0 + k_{OH}[OH^-]$

The phenols (pK_a of about 10) are better leaving groups than aliphatic alcohols like methanol (pK_a about 16), and thus phenol esters are in general hydrolyzed much faster than aliphatic alcohols.

8.13:

$$\begin{array}{ccc}
TC & \underset{k_{-1}}{\overset{k_1}{\rightleftarrows}} & ETC \\
\Big\downarrow k_3 & & \Big\downarrow k_4 \\
ATC & \underset{k_{-2}}{\overset{k_2}{\rightleftarrows}} & EATC
\end{array}$$

The following rate equations are involved:

A: $\dfrac{d[TC]}{dt} = k_{-1}[ETC] - (k_1 + k_3)[TC]$

B: $\dfrac{d[ETC]}{dt} = k_1[TC] - (k_{-1} + k_4)[ETC]$

C: $\dfrac{d[ATC]}{dt} = k_3[TC] + k_{-2}[EATC] - k_2[ATC]$

D: $\dfrac{d[EATC]}{dt} = k_2[ATC] + k_4[ETC] - k_{-2}[EATC]$

We will only use equations A and B to solve the problem. If we assume that the concentration of ETC remains constant (see Chapter 2, section 2.6.4 Steady-state approximation), then:

$$\frac{d[ETC]}{dt} = 0 = k_1[TC] - (k_{-1} + k_4)[ETC] \quad \text{or}$$

$$[ETC] = \frac{k_1}{k_{-1} + k_4}[TC].$$

Substitution into A gives

$$\frac{d[TC]}{dt} = k_{-1}\frac{k_1}{k_{-1} + k_4}[TC] - (k_1 + k_3)[TC]$$

$$= \left[\frac{k_1 k_{-1}}{k_{-1} + k_4} - (k_1 + k_3)\right][TC] = k_{obs}[TC]$$

$$k_{obs} = \frac{k_1 k_{-1}}{k_{-1} + k_4} - (k_1 + k_3)$$

$$= \frac{0.414\ h^{-1} \times 0.373\ h^{-1}}{0.373\ h^{-1} + 0.206\ h^{-1}} - (0.414\ h^{-1} + 0.323\ h^{-1}) = -0.470\ h^{-1}$$

This will give us a simple first-order equation (see Eq. 2.12):

$$-\frac{d[TC]}{dt} = 0.470\ h^{-1}[TC]$$

The shelf-life (t_{90}) can then be calculated according to Eq. 2.19:

$$t_{90} = \frac{0.105}{k_0} = \frac{0.105}{0.470\ h^{-1}} = 0.22\ h = 13.4\ min\ at\ pH\ 1.5\ and\ 60°C.$$

8.14:

This is a question of finding optimal pH for solubility (>200 mg/ml) and stability. The problem can be solved as follows.

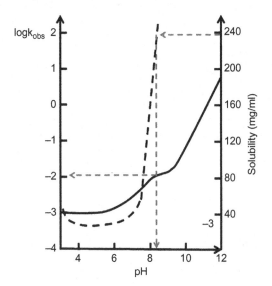

The solubility of the drug in the parenteral formulation has to be greater than 200 mg/ml to prevent drug precipitation due to, for example, pH fluctuations and solvent evaporation. At pH 8.3, the solubility of the drug is about 240 mg/ml. However, at this pH the shelf-life at 25°C is:

$$t_{90} = \frac{0.105}{k_0} \approx \frac{0.105}{1.0 \times 10^{-2}h^{-1}} = 10.5\,h$$

Applying the Q_{10} method to estimate the shelf-life in a refrigerator (5°C), shows that it is less than one week at pH 8.3. The drug has maximum stability at a pH between 3 and 6, but even at that pH it is very unstable ($t_{90} \approx 4$ days at 25°C and less than two months at 5°C). Due to its instability, the drug has to be marketed as lyophilized powder for reconstitution of parenteral solution. Furthermore, due to its low aqueous solubility at acidic and neutral pHs, the pH of the reconstituted solution has to be greater than 8, preferably greater than 8.3. For example, the sodium salt of the drug (β-lactam antibiotic) can be used, and Na_2CO_3 can be included in the lyophilized powder for pH adjustment. Once reconstituted, the solution should not be stored for longer than a couple of hours at room temperature.

REFERENCES

1. S.A. Ranadive, J.D. Pipkin, S.A. Varia, N.H. Chang, E.P. Barry, M. Porubcan, et al., Formation, isolation and identification of oligomers of aztreonam, Eur. J. Pharm. Sci. 3 (1995) 281–291.

2. J.D. de Vries, J. Winkelhorst, W.J.M. Underberg, R.E.C. Henrar, J.H. Beijnen, A systematic study on the chemical stability of the novel indoloquinone antitumour agent EO9, Int. J. Pharm. 100 (1993) 181–188.

Printed in the United States
By Bookmasters